Doctors' Guide to
Chronic
PAIN

Doctors' Guide to
Chronic
PAIN

THE NEWEST, QUICKEST, AND MOST EFFECTIVE WAYS TO FIND

RELIEF

Richard Laliberte

Reader's Digest

The Reader's Digest Association, Inc., Pleasantville, New York/Montreal

READER'S DIGEST PROJECT STAFF

Senior Editor
Nancy Shuker

Senior Designer
Judith Carmel

Production Technology Manager
Douglas A. Croll

Manufacturing Manager
John L. Cassidy

CONTRIBUTORS

Writers
Richard Laliberte
Rachelle Vander Schaaf

Designer
Andrew Ploski

Copy Editor
Jeanette Gingold

Indexer
Nanette Bendyna

MEDICAL EDITOR

Michael R. Clark, MD., M.P.H.
Associate Professor & Director
Chronic Pain Treatment Programs
Dept. of Psychiatry & Behavioral Sciences
The Johns Hopkins Medical Institutions

READER'S DIGEST HEALTH PUBLISHING

Editor-in-Chief
Neil Wertheimer

Design Director
Michele Laseau

Marketing Director
James H. Malloy

Vice President and General Manager
Keira Krausz

READER'S DIGEST ASSOCIATION, INC.

Editor-in-Chief
Eric W. Schrier

President, North American Books and Home Entertainment
Thomas D. Gardner

Library of Congress Cataloging-in-Publication Data

Laliberte, Richard.
    Doctors' guide to chronic pain : the the newest, quickest, and most effective ways to find relief/Richard Laliberte.
        p. cm.
    Includes index.
    ISBN 0-7621-0468-6 (hc)
     1. Chronic pain--Popular works. I. Title: Guide to chronic pain. II Title

    RB127 L275 2003
    616'.0472--dc21

                      2003041279

Address comments about *Doctors' Guide to Chronic Pain* to:
Reader's Digest
Editor-in-Chief, Reader's Digest Health Publishing
Reader's Digest Road, Pleasantville, NY 10570

To order copies of *Doctors' Guide to Chronic Pain*,
call 1-800-846-2100

Visit our website at rd.com

Printed in the United States of America
1 3 5 7 9 10 8 6 4 2 (hardcover)

Note to Readers
The information in this book should not be substituted for, or used to alter, medical therapy without your doctor's advice. For a specific health problem, consult your physician for guidance.

US 4251 H/G

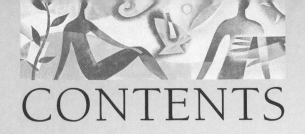

CONTENTS

INTRODUCTION

Patients with chronic pain often find themselves in a world apart. Trapped in a maze of doctors, insurance companies, case managers, and, sometimes, even quacks, they become isolated from family and friends. Struggling to find relief, chronic pain patients can lose the parts of their lives that are most meaningful and enjoyable. This book presents a rational, comprehensive, and optimistic approach to living despite the burden of chronic pain. The message is simple. Patients with chronic pain do not have to suffer—not in silence nor with cries of agony. Modern medicine may not have all the answers but it does have a formidable arsenal of anti-pain weapons to deploy in a variety of ways. The trick is finding the most effective ones for each patient and developing a comprehensive treatment plan—based on earlier failures and more recent successes—that makes sense and offers hope.

Several problems exist in the current approach to chronic pain. Right from the start, the ABC's are sometimes neglected. The basic steps of taking your history, examining you, and formulating an individual diagnosis are truncated. Instead, you can arrive in a doctor's office labeled "chronic pain patient" and the doctor won't bother with a customized diagnosis, but just prescribe a standard treatment. What the doctor misses is your unique nature, your individual diagnosis, and the potential to develop a specific treatment regimen designed just for you. In other words, this reductionistic approach to chronic pain results in shotgun medicine. Treatments are prescribed without specific targets.

On the other hand, if your doctor gets hung up on finding a diagnosis for your unexplained pain, treatment may again be sacrificed. A patient with chronic pain is often subjected to inconvenient, expensive, risky, and painful attempts to discover the cause of the pain. This search can be all-consuming. Meanwhile, you can lose function, become depressed, exhaust your personal resources, and, finally, move to another doctor. Eventually, no one really knows your case. When this process repeats itself and no progress is made, a vicious cycle is born.

Another problem in the treatment of chronic pain arises from your doctor's recognition that a cure for your condition is unlikely and your pain may really prove to be chronic. Your doctor may stop trying and start to focus on not rocking the boat, keeping the situation from getting worse, and hoping you will settle down with your pain. Your doctor may stop using aggressive treatments and trying new alternatives. You, like many patients, may settle down in discouragement or start looking for a different doctor. You will be justified in feeling abandoned by your doctor..

Recognizing that the management of pain care in modern medicine is finally improving, the advice for chronic pain patients presented in this book is organized around several important themes.

First, expect more. Patients with chronic pain should never settle for less than full attention to their problems from the medical profession. The goal of treatment is to alleviate all the manifestations of their illness and to return to them all the benefits of health. In short, no pain and full function. While this may be difficult to attain, the striving for success will force reassessment, modification, and creativity in an ongoing process of treatment that keeps the relationship between patient and doctors strong.

Second, be active. Patients with chronic pain cannot afford to be passive. Waiting for relief to be provided won't help you regain control of your life. Take charge and do something for yourself. Chronic pain is certainly a burden to be shouldered, but it need not be an anchor to tie you down. Patients should think constantly about their situation and how they can improve it. Asking questions – what do we know? what did we learn? how did that help us? – keeps the focus on problem solving and coping.

Finally, stay optimistic. Pessimism and hopelessness are not the inevitable outcomes of chronic pain. New research, new techniques, new medications, and new equipment are constantly being produced. Each one offers hope and opportunity for improvement.

Even now, the combinations for designing treatment plans are unlimited. There is always something else to try, a next step to work toward.

MICHAEL R. CLARK, M.D., M.P.H.
Dr. Clark, chief medical consultant for this book, is Associate Professor & Director for Chronic Pain Treatment Programs, Department of Psychiatry & Behavioral Sciences at The Johns Hopkins Medical Institutions in Baltimore.

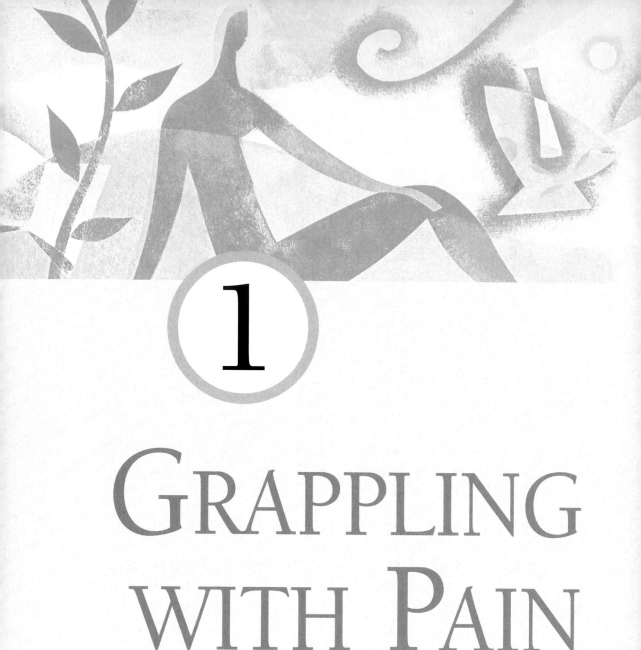

1

GRAPPLING WITH PAIN

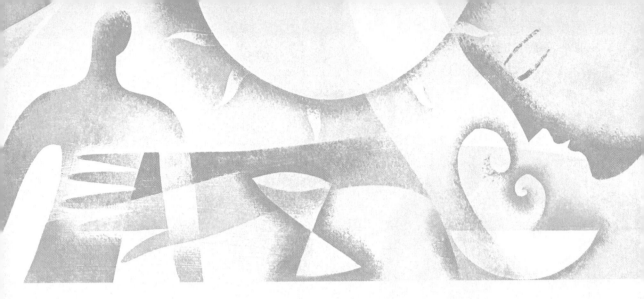

For patients who must live with chronic pain, the modern medical profession's new attitude toward their suffering should come as welcome news. Recognition of pain as a factor to be reckoned with has changed the way that doctors treat chronic diseases and has sped up research into pain-relieving medications and procedures. Patients, too, have changed and are learning to ask for the help they need—and deserve—to overcome their discomfort and disabilities.

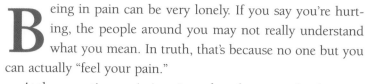

Being in pain can be very lonely. If you say you're hurting, the people around you may not really understand what you mean. In truth, that's because no one but you can actually "feel your pain."

At the same time, pain is universal, and on some level, everyone can relate to it. Ultimately, relief of suffering is the reason we have medicine, and doctors have traditionally fulfilled this healing mandate by trying to fix the problems that lead to pain and discomfort. It's not a misguided approach: You'll find valuable information on alleviating pain from a range of important chronic conditions later in this book.

But there's a drawback to concentrating solely on medical conditions: It often relegates pain to being "merely" a symptom of an underlying disease—an indicator of what's going wrong, but not a problem worth serious scrutiny and treatment on its own. Fortunately, though, that point of view is beginning to change as researchers delve deeper into the mysteries of pain. Scientists are finding that pain's causes are complex, its effects can be stubbornly persistent and that, left untreated, it can often acquire a torturous life of its own. "It used to be assumed that there was a direct relationship between [disease or injury] pathology and pain, but the fact is, you can't always identify a pathology," says pain researcher Dennis C. Turk, Ph.D., professor of anesthesiology at the University of Washington in Seattle. "That doesn't mean you're faking it." In many chronic cases, pain seems to be the disease.

The fact that pain can't be objectively detected or measured—"there's no pain thermometer," says Turk—has made doctors in the past leery of self-reported suffering. Patients who complained about pain were often suspected of exaggerating, especially when a physical cause wasn't obvious. As a result, pain was (and still is) often undertreated.

Although pain management advocates say far more still must be done, today pain is often seen as a condition worth addressing solely on the basis of a patient's say-so. That's good news for the more than 50 million Americans who suffer from chronic pain, as well as the 25 million more who experience acute pain every year due to injuries or surgery.

If you're among the miserable, you may not welcome the

company—but you can take comfort in how the scope of the problem has helped spur some significant developments:

- **Pain management recognition.** Pain management is becoming—slowly—a recognized medical specialty with stand-alone centers, clinics treating specific conditions, and pain management departments in hospitals.

- **The "fifth vital sign."** Professional societies and advocacy groups—the American Pain Society, the American Pain Foundation, the American Academy of Pain Medicine, and the American Academy of Pain Management—have sprung up to nudge the medical establishment into paying more attention to pain. The idea that pain is the "fifth vital sign," along with temperature, pulse, respiration, and blood pressure, to indicate the overall state of a person's health is gaining wider acceptance.

- **The medical establishment is listening.** Case in point: The Joint Commission on the Accreditation of Healthcare Organizations (JCAHO) recently introduced new standards that require hospitals, nursing homes, and other health facilities to assess and control pain. Failure to do so is now considered not only unethical but medically unsound, because pain by itself often leads to future health problems that harm patients and waste healthcare resources. Facilities that skimp on pain control can now be threatened with losing their accreditation.

- **Successful research for more effective pain-relief drugs.** For example, an entirely new class of anti-inflammatory medications called COX-2 inhibitors (e.g., Celebrex and Vioxx) became available in the late 1990s; a new drug of this class (Bextra) joined the ranks in mid-2002.

- **A new view of complementary alternative medicine.** Doctors are becoming more open to alternative therapies such as acupuncture that show promise for relieving certain kinds of pain. While research on alternative medicine is often inconclusive, doctors are becoming less resistant to unconventional methods if patients say the therapies provide relief.

- **Legal help.** Legislation is being passed at both the state and federal levels to support and define guidelines for treating pain.

PAIN STATISTICS

Despite progress, pain care in the U.S. is far from satisfactory. Some telling statistics from *The Journal of the American Medical Association* and other sources:

> Patients receive adequate care for acute pain in only one of four U.S. surgeries.

> Forty percent of people with moderate to severe chronic pain can't get satisfactory relief.

> Only about 30 percent of cancer patients get adequate relief of their pain.

> Only a quarter of people with moderate to severe chronic pain ever get a referral to a pain specialist.

Your Right to Relief

Although considerable progress has been made in pain management, the American Pain Foundation still maintains that "finding good pain care and taking control of your pain can be hard work." The fact is, doctors don't always give pain control the priority they should. Alleviating pain is basic to your healthcare, however, and you have a right to insist on getting the best relief possible.

To protect yourself, you need to know how pain works, how it can be treated, what care you have a right to expect, and what may be preventing you from getting the care you need. Many doctors and nurses who specialize in pain control lament the fact that in an age of biotechnology, genetic engineering, organ transplants, and sophisticated surgery, pain—the common denominator—is still given less attention than it deserves among rank-and-file medical professionals.

WHAT CAN COMPROMISE YOUR CARE

Why would doctors, whose avowed goal is to cure disease, relieve suffering, restore the benefits of health, improve the quality of life, and—above all—avoid doing harm, fail to adequately manage pain when it's evident in patients right in front of their noses? There are several possible reasons:

Lack of training. Although the field of pain management is growing, fewer than one percent of doctors are trained pain specialists. Most doctors receive little clinical or classroom instruction on pain management, which is still seen as less important than other fundamentals of care, such as, say, the biology of blood clotting or the basics of childbirth. In fact, while aspiring doctors must pass stiff examinations for obstetrics and gynecology (OB-GYN), which potentially affects half of patients (women), there are no such requirements for pain management, which potentially affects all patients (men and women). Seeing that pain management gets low priority among their teachers and peers, many doctors pay little attention to it in training or in practice.

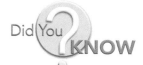

Did You KNOW

Pain has often been viewed as a form of divine retribution for mortal misdeeds (as in God cursing Eve to experience childbirth pain after eating the forbidden fruit). Theologians today generally don't interpret suffering as direct spiritual castigation, but the idea is embedded in our language: The word "pain" comes from the Latin poena, which means "punishment."

Biases. In much of the medical community pain management is not yet as respected as other specialties. And in some areas of medicine, empathy is not encouraged for fear that doctors who are too close to their patients' suffering will lose their clinical objectivity.

Conservative outlook. For medically sound reasons, doctors tend to be a cautious bunch. Often, they'll hesitate to prescribe a drug (especially a narcotic) unless there's a clear and obvious need for it. They prefer to start with less-powerful drugs at the least potent doses over the longest period of time they can justify. This is not necessarily wrong: If low doses of weak drugs do the job, there's no need to bring out bigger cannons. But if you don't know heavier weaponry waits in the wings, you might assume your doctor has already done everything possible. And you may be reluctant to "complain" or tell the doctor that you're still in pain.

Expediency. In a perfect world, practical considerations like time and money wouldn't affect quality of care, but in contemporary life they sometimes do. In purely pragmatic terms, pain management takes time—to talk, assess, diagnose, prescribe, follow up—and adds a level of complexity to patient care. In the

THE PAIN-RELIEF PLEDGE

Pain-care standards agreed to by hospitals, nursing homes, and other healthcare facilities certified by the Joint Commission on the Accreditation of Healthcare Organizations (JCAHO) include the following principles—important steps toward improving pain management practices:

✴ Patients have a right to have their pain assessed and managed, and healthcare facilities should communicate their commitment to pain care through mission statements, a patient bill of rights, or publicly stated service standards.

✴ Every patient should be asked about pain—whether you have any, what its nature is, and how intense it is. Healthcare organizations should have standard procedures for making these assessments, recording results, and following up on them—especially when patients leave the facility. What's more, clinical staff should be trained in pain assessment and management, and be evaluated on how well they actually do it.

✴ It's just as important to treat symptoms like pain as it is to treat underlying diseases or conditions, and patients in pain should be given appropriate pain-relieving medication.

✴ Patients and their families should be educated about how important pain management is to overall care. Fear of opioid drugs—common in patients and physicians—should be addressed with accurate information that dispels misconceptions.

✴ Pain management should be part of an organization's own performance quality assessments, and changes should be considered if performance data suggest they're needed.

competitive pressure cooker that healthcare has become in some settings, these are not incentives for doctors to pay more attention to pain, especially when doing so brings little in the way of extra reimbursement.

Fear. Patients may be reluctant to bring up pain, for fear it will distract their doctor from treating the disease. And because treating pain with medication often involves prescription of opioid (narcotic) drugs, many doctors are afraid they'll run afoul of the law if patients abuse their pain relievers or become addicted to them. Such worries are largely unfounded: There's little risk of addiction in patients who take opioids in dosages adequate for pain relief. Still, news reports of doctors being arrested for supplying drugs to unscrupulous patients stir doctors' (and many patients') concerns. Remember that you and your doctor are partners in your care

KNOW YOUR RIGHTS

Pain management advocates say individual doctors will become more motivated to deal with patient pain when they sense greater grassroots pressure to do so—from you and other sufferers. That doesn't mean you have to march in the streets, petition the hospital board, or personally lobby Capitol Hill. Instead, consider your doctor your ally and talk calmly and candidly with her or him about your needs and concerns. Remember that you and your doctor are partners in your care.

According to the American Pain Foundation, you have a right to expect—and, if need be, demand—that:

- **Your pain be thoroughly assessed** and promptly treated.
- **Your doctor keep you informed** about what might be causing your pain, how it might be treated, how treatment could help you, and what the costs and risks of each treatment would be.
- **You actively participate** in decisions about how to manage your pain.
- **Your pain is reassessed** regularly and your treatment adjusted if you're not getting satisfactory relief.
- **You get clear and prompt answers** to questions, and get the time you need to make decisions.
- **You are able to refuse** a specific treatment if you want.
- **You get a referral** to a pain specialist if your pain persists.

An Action Plan for Pain

Dealing with chronic pain can make you feel helpless, a passive victim of forces beyond your command. But while pain can't always be completely eliminated, there's much you can do to take charge of your own relief. By taking action, you gain a feeling of control. That alone provides comfort for many people suffering from persistent pain.

Effective pain relief starts with you. You may be surrounded by caring people—your doctor, your family, your friends—who want to ease your pain. They can help you in many ways, but taking control is ultimately what you must do for yourself. Even if pain continues to nag you, you don't have to let it rule your life. You can gain empowerment over pain with the following action plan:

① **Get help.** This may seem obvious—everybody sees a doctor to alleviate pain. The trick is to continue seeking help if your doctor can't provide you with the relief you need. This isn't necessarily a failure of will on your doctor's part: Pain is a nefarious and elusive enemy that can hide its true nature even from experienced physicians. At the same time, it's easy to feel that continuing to report pain after a doctor has prescribed a remedy makes you the problem—a complainer who becomes a thorn in the physician's side. Don't get drawn into this kind of thinking. Good doctors recognize that they don't always have all the answers, and will either seek new approaches on their own or refer you to someone who may be able to help you more. Don't be afraid to ask for the further relief you have a right to expect if you feel you need it. Work on communicating with your doctor so that you can be candid. This is a special relationship—not so much as friendship as a partnership in treating your illness—and it deserves nurturing.

② **Address the underlying problem**. While chronic pain can be mysterious, it's not inexplicable. Your pain does have a cause—even if it's not obvious—and the more persistently you and your doctor work to find it, the easier it will be to design an effective treatment. In many cases, pain has its roots in a known injury or disease such as one of the various forms of arthritis or a jolt to the lower back. In other cases, the problem is rooted in the nervous system. Often, resolving an underlying condition alone can ease the suffering. But doctors who study how pain works also use an approach called "mechanism-based diagnosis," in which knowledge of the ways pain registers in the brain can help direct therapy.

③ **Form a plan.** The more involved you are with decisions about your pain management, the better you'll feel about it—and

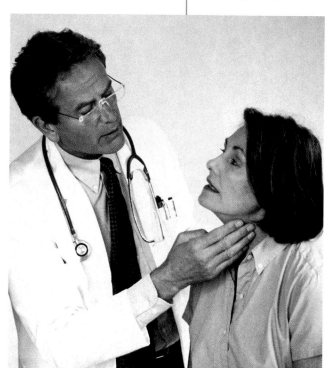

the more effective your treatment is likely to be. Studies find that when arthritis patients actively participate in their care, for example, they experience less pain, pay fewer visits to the doctor, and—most important—enjoy life more. Start by keeping records about your pain—how it feels, when it pops up, what activities aggravate it—and learn as much as you can about your underlying condition or the possible pathways that may be causing your pain. Then work with your doctor to develop a program to move you past your pain. Together, decide on reasonable quality-of-life goals that you can work toward, whether it's going back to work, getting a decent night's sleep, enjoying sex again, or participating in a favorite sport. Don't be too ambitious at the beginning. Start with small goals you can easily achieve to keep from becoming discouraged.

④ **Ask about medication.** Once you've agreed on goals, work with your doctor to clearly lay out the treatments you'll be using, especially medications. Be sure you understand each drug's benefits and any side effects that may result from its use. If you don't understand, be sure to ask questions. If your doctor isn't prescribing drugs for you, ask why not—especially if other forms of therapy aren't helping.

(5) **Look beyond drugs.** While pain medications can go a long way toward relieving suffering, you can't rely on them entirely—and fortunately (because they often have unpleasant side effects such as nausea, lethargy, or gastrointestinal irritation, depending on what you use) you don't have to. Don't be surprised if your doctor actually suggests you start with non-drug pain management methods such as relaxation therapy, exercise, physical therapy, heat and cold, massage, or other treatments. Many doctors, in fact, feel the main purpose drugs fulfill is to take the edge off pain well enough to allow movement-based treatments, especially exercise and physical therapy. In many cases, the most effective pain-relief program will involve the use of several treatment methods at once.

(6) **Recognize the power within.** Researchers increasingly realize that pain involves a close interaction between mind and body, and that emotions, personal values, interpretation, context and meaning all can affect how we experience pain. While the interplay of mind and body is complex, it's become clear that you can use the inner power of your mind to control—or at least change—the intensity or quality of pain, even if the pain doesn't entirely go away. That's good news for chronic pain sufferers because it's opened the door to a range of "thought therapies" that can provide significant comfort without further use of medications and their side effects.

(7) **Explore alternatives.** Perhaps because pain management specialists recognize the legitimate benefits of mind/body therapies (which science-based Western medicine has traditionally regarded with skepticism), they've also led the medical community in trying complementary alternative medicine (CAM). This approach uses alternative methods of pain relief in conjunction with traditional medicine. Doctors who recommend these alternatives don't contend that every form of complementary medicine is legitimate. But they do suggest that some CAM approaches to pain relief may be worth exploring. Unorthodox methods such as acupunc-

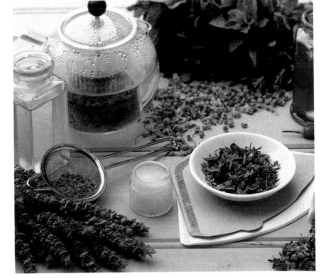

MYTHS ABOUT PAIN

Pain is tough enough to manage without worrying about "facts" that aren't grounded in reality but can nevertheless drag you down. Among the noxious (and unhelpful) beliefs about pain:

I just have to live with it.
The fact is, most pain can be relieved or significantly eased with proper pain management, according to the American Pain Foundation.

If I can't take it, I must be weak.
Actually, people have different tolerances for pain based on a wide variety of factors, including the physical mechanisms of pain, psychological variables, and even cultural influences—all of which may be beyond your control. Your pain is what it is and is not a reflection on your character.

Once pain starts, I can't stop it. Pain can sometimes magnify itself—but it's not a process beyond your control. The more you do to manage your discomfort, the less likely it is that your pain will get worse. If pain medications have been prescribed for you, take them at the first sign of trouble and call your doctor if pain becomes more agonizing.

If I take drugs, I'll get hooked.
The majority of prescription pain relievers are not habit-forming. Those that are (e.g, opioid medications such as morphine) aren't likely to cause addiction if your doctor prescribes them properly and you take them as directed.

I shouldn't complain.
Neither should you tough it out. Remember that pain control starts with you. You can't be helped if you don't make your needs known.

ture, biofeedback, and therapeutic touch, for example, hold promise for relief without seeming to carry significant risks.

⑧ Manage your emotions. Chronic physical pain quickly becomes psychic pain as well, dredging up malignant emotions such as depression, anxiety, and anger—all of which conspire to make your pain even worse. Research into the neurology of pain shows that the signals for pain and emotion share common pathways through the nervous system, suggesting that dark emotions can contribute to triggering pain. That makes it doubly important that you do everything you can—from talk therapy and antidepressants to combination treatments that take advantage of both—to treat mental illnesses associated with your pain.

⑨ Enlist support. Yes, you're in charge of your care because no one has a better sense of your needs and goals (and your determination to address them) than you. But you don't have to fight your battle against pain by yourself. Having a strong network of family and friends to help you cope has tangible benefits beyond the enjoyment you may feel from being around others. In fact, people with strong social support tend to cope better with chronic pain, feel less depressed, retain greater independence, and enjoy a range of other boosts to well-being such as stronger immune function and longer life. Chronic pain can make communication with others more difficult, and strain even healthy bonds—unless you take steps to consciously develop and nurture the relationships that are most important to you. Keep up the interests that you share with family and friends and stay in touch.

⑩ **Never give up.** Perhaps the most difficult aspect of chronic pain to deal with is the fact that it doesn't let up. This can make your relief-seeking efforts—and when things really seem bad, your life itself—seem hopeless and perhaps even not worth continuing. Doctors know this and are aiming their efforts at the intersection of hope and medicine. "If a doctor says, 'Pain is a problem we can correct. Here's something you can try,' that's very different than saying, 'I can't find anything wrong,' " Turk says. "If you feel helpless, you'll perceive pain as more intense. But if you feel in control, it will feel less intense." In the interests of providing patients with greater control, pain management understanding and techniques continue to improve—and that's reason for hope.

What Is Pain?

It seems an odd question to ask when virtually every person on earth can provide an answer from experience. But that's just the problem: All of us have our own definition and history of pain, and its highly subjective nature can be tough to pin down. Fortunately, although much remains to be learned, we live at a time when science actually has some answers about the sometimes baffling nature of pain.

It's important to learn as much as you can about how pain works, because better understanding will make your action plan more effective, your consultations with your doctor more meaningful, and your sense of control over your suffering sharper. In the art of war (and you are definitely in a battle—with a daunt-

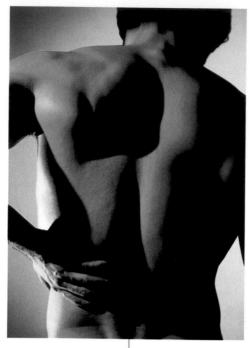

ing adversary), the first step toward victory is getting to know the enemy.

Start by considering the definition of pain that doctors tend to fall back on from the International Association for the Study of Pain, a leading research organization. The IASP says pain is "an unpleasant sensory and emotional experience associated with actual or potential tissue damage, or described in terms of such damage." It's a definition that deliberately leaves the door open to a variety of possibilities.

"Pain isn't just one thing," says Perry Fine, M.D., professor of anesthesiology and director of the Pain Management Center at the University of Utah School of Medicine in Salt Lake City. The most important part of the IASP definition may be its emphasis on pain as both a sensory and an emotional experience. "Those two aspects of pain simply can't be separated," says Fine. But the IASP also notes how pain can be complex in other ways as well. "For example, pain is often based on injury—but it doesn't have to be," says Fine. "If I press a tender point at the base of your neck, that's not causing an injury, but it still hurts." In this example, the pain is associated with a potential injury—because if the pressing on your shoulder continues to get harder, it will eventually cause physical harm.

THE BOTTOM LINE: When you're in pain, it feels like your body or health is being damaged or threatened, which is likely to provoke a strong emotional response.

PAIN IN PERSPECTIVE

It may be a small consolation when you're hurting, but pain is supposed to be good for us. In fact, it plays an important role in keeping us healthy—and even saving our lives. "Initially, pain is a survival mechanism," says Fine. As the IASP suggests by linking pain to potential injury, we're designed to react to pain in order to avoid further harm. Without pain, you'd never jerk your hand back from touching a hot stove, nurse a cut on the bottom of your foot, or learn to avoid foods that don't agree with your gut. People who suffer from a rare disorder that leaves them impervious to pain often die young because they aren't able to detect their injuries. More commonly, people with diabetes who suffer from nerve damage, a common complication, can have trouble feeling injuries to their feet, often resulting in permanent damage that makes diabetes the leading cause of lower-limb amputations in the U.S.

At the same time, for pain to truly promote well-being, it has to have limits. The skin, which is intricately wired with millions of sensory nerve endings, can pick up all kinds of extremely delicate signals that could conceivably suggest possible injury, but we can't afford to interpret every touch of a butterfly's wings as pain. As a result, we tend to be selective about the sensations and pains we pay attention to, and the amount of pain we can tolerate sometimes changes based on what' else is happening to us or giving us trouble at the time.

Given this balance of sensation, how and why the body experiences pain has been a source of rich speculation for centuries. In the ancient world, pain was attributed to demons or dead spirits, or (as Plato suggested) the intrusion of "particles" into

WHEN PAIN MAY BE AN EMERGENCY

Even if your attention is focused on chronic pain, you shouldn't ignore acute pains that may signal a serious new condition. Seek medical help immediately if you experience any of the following:

PAIN	POSSIBLE CAUSE
Unusual sudden, intense headache.	If your speech, vision or thinking is also affected, or if you experience partial paralysis (especially on one side of the body), you may be suffering from a stroke. If the headache is accompanied by fever, vomiting, drowsiness, or a stiff neck, you could have meningitis, a type of brain infection.
Chest pain that may be accompanied by pain or numbness in the face, arms, neck or back, as well as shortness of breath, sweating, dizziness, or nausea.	You could be having a heart attack or other cardiovascular-related problems such as an aneurysm (an abnormal dilation of a blood vessel wall) or an embolism (a type of blood vessel obstruction).
Severe abdominal pain.	If pain spreads over your lower right side, you could have appendicitis; your lower left side, diverticulitis. If cramping is accompanied by bloating, nausea, or vomiting, or if you have trouble passing solid waste or gas, you could have an intestinal obstruction. If you have difficulty voiding or see blood in your urine, you could have kidney stones.
Sudden, painful swelling and inflammation of a joint, especially in one or both knees.	Could be the result of an injury, but if you also experience fever and chills, you could have some form of arthritis.

the soul. One of the most important theories—both for what it got right and what it got wrong—was developed by René Descartes, the famous 17th-century philosopher, mathematician, and scientist. Descartes astutely suggested that pain was different from ordinary touch, and was processed through a network of filaments connecting the skin and the brain. When you hurt yourself, Descartes said, pain rings an alarm in your head like a rope pulling a bell.

TWO TYPES OF PAIN

Descartes' vision of the anatomy of pain remains a helpful—but incomplete—way to think about how the message is transmitted. His ideas about pain, however, didn't go very far in distinguishing between different types of pain. In current practice, doctors and patients alike recognize that, while pain can be categorized in a variety of ways, there are two basic forms of pain—acute and chronic.

Acute pain. You can think of acute pain as "healthy" pain—the immediate, get-your-attention, save-yourself type of pain familiar to anyone who's been cut, bruised, lacerated, scraped, hit, burned, or had a bone broken. As a rule, you have a clear understanding of whatever is causing acute pain, whether it's a surgical incision, an aching tooth, a boil, or childbirth. It's also generally clear how long acute pain can be expected to last—for example, until the stitches heal, the root canal is over, the swelling subsides, or the baby has been happily delivered. Acute pain acts like any other form of touch—for example, if you press the painful area, it will hurt more—and it serves a purpose. Although it can last for days, and perhaps even months, acute pain is marked by generally being short-lived, predictable, and restricted to a specific area—characteristics that some researchers refer to as "physiological pain."

Chronic pain. Consider chronic pain the evil twin of acute pain: The two types can seem alike on the surface, but chronic pain is a vicious malingerer. One basic difference between acute and chronic pain is simple duration: Chronic pain tends to go on and on, and is usually defined as

SUBDIVIDING SUFFERING

While pain is fundamentally divided into acute and chronic categories, there are many ways of classifying different types of painful experience. Some classifications are based on where pain originates, while others are based on how pain behaves:

Breakthrough pain
Pain that flares up despite your taking analgesic medication.

Intermittent pain
Pain that comes and goes, or increases and decreases in intensity, but doesn't seem to leave for good.

Musculoskeletal pain
Aching in the muscles, bones, or joints, a broad category of pain that includes arthritis, back and neck pain, fibromyalgia, and headaches.

Neuropathic pain
Pain that results from damage to the nerves themselves (among its causes are diabetes, cancer, and unintended harm from surgery), often producing sharp tingling or burning sensations.

Trigger-point pain
Sometimes called myofascial pain, it's characterized by extreme tenderness in small areas of muscle that can often refer pain to other parts of the body.

Visceral pain
Pain arising from the viscera, or internal organs. It's usually associated with abdominal problems and is often described as a dull aching.

occurring daily for six months or more. But chronic pain is more than a long-lasting version of acute pain. The source of chronic pain can be maddeningly difficult to pinpoint. What's more, it generally outlives any connection it may have had to actual physical harm and may, in fact, get worse for no apparent reason. Because chronic pain serves no biological purpose, it's no longer pain that's good for you. In fact, it becomes a problem all its own—what researchers sometimes call "pathophysiological" or "clinical" pain.

How Pain Works

The basic way pain registers physically within the body seems simple: Some type of "noxious stimulus" (to use the parlance of pain research) in a particular part of the body sends a signal to the brain through the nervous system and makes you say "ouch." But that only begins to describe the pain process, which involves two-way messaging that allows the brain to talk back to the body.

Pain encompasses a cascade of signals involving not only nerves, but a range of chemicals, enzymes, and other substances in the body that engage each other in amazingly diverse ways. It may be fortunate that pain is as intricate as it is because many steps along its pathway offer the potential for the process to be altered through a spectrum of soothing therapies.

THE PROCESS OF PAIN

Pain is so important to the body that nature has provided a class of sensory nerve endings whose sole job is to register pain messages and forward them to the brain. Called nociceptors (from the Latin words *nocere* and *recipere,* which mean "hurt" and "receive"), these nerve endings are found by the millions throughout the body, but are heavily concentrated in the skin and muscles. That's why we tend to feel pain more intensely in those areas than, say, the insides of our organs or the outsides of our bones. When you cut your finger or stub your toe (injury-prone areas especially rich in nociceptors), activated

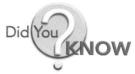

The cerebral cortex of the brain is wired to receive greater input from some areas of the body than others—part of the reason certain parts of the anatomy are more sensitive to pain. Among the regions the brain's circuits are most densely programmed to perceive are your mouth and lips, face, head, hands, and big toes.

nerve endings pass the word along through a number of different nerve pathways—a process known as nociception. Not all nerve endings are created equal, but instead are assigned specialized sensations, with some registering sharp, stinging feelings, and others sensing, say, temperature, pressure, or inflammation.

Interestingly, nerves don't move all pain signals along with equal speed. Some signals, like sharp pains, zip to the brain almost instantly, while others, such as dull and persistent aches, travel more slowly. That's why a cut in your finger or a blow to your toe first smarts, then starts to throb a moment later.

Pain signals follow a number of different pathways through the nervous system that enable the body to respond in a variety of ways. For example, some fast-moving signals dash off to motor nerves that make you quickly jerk your foot off a sharp object or your finger from a hot stove. Other signals may ring the body's stress alarm, triggering the release of hormones like cortisol and epinephrine, which prepare your body to take action against danger by boosting your heart rate, raising blood pressure, increasing your respiration, and pumping sugar into your blood. Still other signals spur inflammation, which, though meant to promote healing, also results in pain.

THE CHEMICAL CONNECTION

How all these signals are ferried through the body is important to understanding pain and the ways it can be managed. In some cases, signals are carried as electrical impulses through the nerves. But the pain response also involves the release of a wide variety of chemicals. These include signal-carrying compounds, or neurotransmitters, such as glutamate, immune system hormones called cytokines, the inflammatory chemical histamine, and a variety of small proteins called peptides. One peptide that seems particularly important, called substance P, appears to make nerves more sensitive to pain.

Many of these chemicals foster inflammation and contribute to the marshaling of prostaglandins, a group of chemicals that play a key role in the pain cascade. Prostaglandins act as short-lived hormones with a range of powerful effects throughout the body. Among other things, they help regulate blood pressure, the female reproductive cycle, fever, and the burning of fat for energy. Most pertinent to pain, however, they also stimulate inflammation; controlling the flood of prostaglandins to the site of damage or injury is how anti-inflammatory drugs like aspirin take the edge off pain.

HIGHWAYS TO THE BRAIN

The brain acts as a central command post in the pain response, both gathering perceptions from the body's peripheries and sending orders back to, say, make the body take immediate action to avoid further harm or gear up the immune system to patch an injury. To get where they're going, pain signals travel a web of nerves that spread throughout the body and feed into the spinal cord. Sometimes compared to the root system of a tree

PAIN PROCESSING STEPS

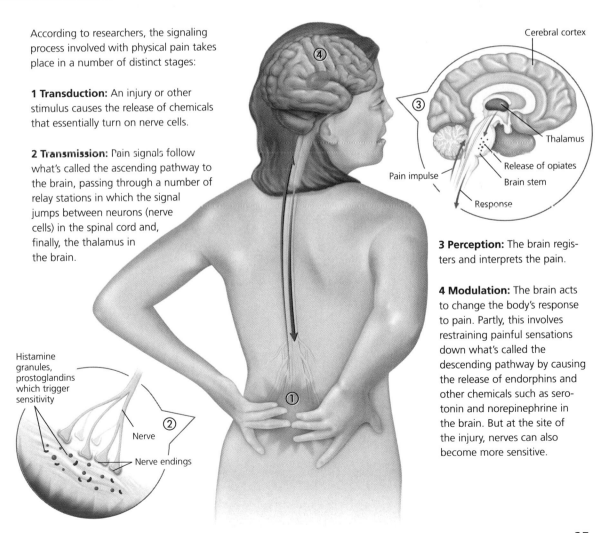

According to researchers, the signaling process involved with physical pain takes place in a number of distinct stages:

1 Transduction: An injury or other stimulus causes the release of chemicals that essentially turn on nerve cells.

2 Transmission: Pain signals follow what's called the ascending pathway to the brain, passing through a number of relay stations in which the signal jumps between neurons (nerve cells) in the spinal cord and, finally, the thalamus in the brain.

Cerebral cortex

Thalamus

Pain impulse

Release of opiates

Brain stem

Response

3 Perception: The brain registers and interprets the pain.

4 Modulation: The brain acts to change the body's response to pain. Partly, this involves restraining painful sensations down what's called the descending pathway by causing the release of endorphins and other chemicals such as serotonin and norepinephrine in the brain. But at the site of the injury, nerves can also become more sensitive.

Histamine granules, prostoglandins which trigger sensitivity

Nerve

Nerve endings

that funnels into the trunk, or a freeway system of ancillary roads that merge into superhighways, nerve signals follow dorsal columns along the back of the spinal cord up to the brain.

In the brain, pain signals go first to the thalamus, the command post's war room, which sorts through messages and acts on them (by triggering reflex actions, for example) or relays them to other parts of the brain. Other stops in the chain of communication include the cerebral cortex, which governs higher thought, and the limbic system, which governs emotion. It's in these areas that pain is analyzed and interpreted. The cerebral cortex, for example, determines where the pain is located and how bad an injury you've sustained. It then uses these judgments to send commands back down to the body to, for example, control blood flow at the site. But both the cerebral cortex and limbic system also contribute to your interpretation of what's happening, which can have a significant impact on how intensely you feel your pain.

DOLING OUT NATURAL PAINKILLERS

The pain process isn't all about noxious stimulation. In fact, once both brain and body understand that pain has registered and action has been taken (danger is being dodged, wounds are being healed), pain becomes less useful as a survival function and steps are taken to keep it in check.

One way this happens is that the brain releases the natural equivalent of opioid drugs into the body from stockpiles in the thalamus, limbic system, hypothalamus (another area of the brain), and spinal cord. Known collectively as endorphins, these hormones were discovered in the 1970s by researchers who were trying to figure out why opioid drugs like morphine had such powerful analgesic effects in the body—and why people sometimes craved them. Scientists first found that brain cells have special "parking places" called receptors designed just for opioids. Then other researchers made the amazing discovery that internal (or endogenous—the word "endorphin" is short for "endogenous morphine") chemicals essentially make the pained brain self-medicating.

Endorphins have since been found to help regulate sex drive, appetite, body temperature, and a range of other functions— including the euphoria that comes from vigorous exercise, sometimes called "runner's high." But their role in pain management appears to be based on their ability to block the communication of pain messages by, for example, suppressing the pain-enhancing release of substance P. So when you're responding to physical pain, think of a fountain of hurtful signals moving up to the brain from the body being met by a waterfall of competing feel-good chemicals coming back down. Signals become muted and jumbled, and the body feels less pain.

CLOSING THE GATE

It was once thought that pain was directly related to how badly damaged your body was—the bigger the injury, the bigger the pain. But anybody who's watched an athlete play through a muscle sprain knows this isn't always true. For years, researchers struggled to explain this paradox. Finally, in the mid-1960s, two researchers (Ronald Melzak and Patrick Wall) proposed what's become known as the gate control theory.

According to this theory (which has been substantiated by more recent pain research), pain signals on their way to the brain pass through a number of junctures that are shared by other types of messages zinging through the nervous system. Because the neural circuitry at these junctures can only handle a limited amount of information, the brain picks and chooses which signals to let through. As a result, competing signals can override pain and essentially close the gate of the pain pathway.

The gateway to pain can be closed in a number of ways. One is for the brain to send the body's own analgesic chemicals to the gateway to prevent pain-related chemicals from doing their jobs. Another is to clutter the nervous system with extra sensory input by, say, rubbing a sore spot or touching it with an ice pack. But just as important, conscious thoughts or sensations completely unrelated to the pain, such as the mental picture of yourself walking on a beach, or listening to a favorite Mozart concerto, can also run interference on pain and make the gate swing further closed.

DOES PAIN MEAN YOU'RE SMART?

Pain cuts across all lines of money and class—but perhaps not intelligence, suggests research at Princeton University.

When scientists genetically engineered a strain of mice that did better on brainpower tests than other mice, they wondered if the smart mice would feel more pain as well. Reason: The scientists had tinkered with a type of molecule called an NMDA receptor, which plays a variety of roles in the central nervous system. In further tests, they found the smarter mice indeed reacted more strongly to chronic—but not acute—pain. While the link between intelligence and pain perception may not apply to humans, scientists say identifying a receptor involved with pain could potentially lead to new drugs for chronic pain.

BARRING THE GATE THEORY

When the gate control theory of pain was first published in 1965, many prominent researchers recognized it for what it was: "Undoubtedly one of the major revolutions in our concept of pain in the last 100 years," as one leader in the field acknowledged at the time. But like any radical idea, it won just as many skeptics among die-hard believers in the specificity theory, the idea that pain was directly related to injury—which dated back to Descartes in the 17th century. While critics who called the theory "unlikely" or "incomplete" were still being heard as recently as the 1980s (and some parts of the initial theory were wrong), the gate control model of pain is now widely accepted.

THE FIBER FACTOR

According to the gate control theory, how much pain you feel also depends to some extent on what type of nerve fibers are carrying the most information at any given time. Motor nerves controlling large muscle movement and nerves that register non-painful touch are all large and conduct their signals relatively quickly compared to pain fibers, which are smaller and conduct messages more slowly. That's one reason why you may not notice pain while you're playing tennis or touch football, but will feel it when you stop.

Why Chronic Pain Is Different

When pain obeys the rules, it follows an understandable pattern—you hurt, you heal, and the pain goes away. So why does pain sometimes continue taking its torturous toll beyond its usefulness as a response to injury? Why can it seem to flare for no apparent physical reason, perhaps in tandem with a bout of depression or anxiety? The answers (to the extent they're known) lie in the brain and nervous system.

One explanation for the persistence of chronic pain is that a pain-causing condition like arthritis simply continues to provide unpleasant stimuli. But pain is more complex than this cause-effect model suggests. It was long assumed that the pain system was a kind of unchanging mechanism that worked according to predictable principles not unlike the electrical wiring in your home. When you turn on a light switch, you don't expect the wires in your walls to start rearranging themselves and forming new connections so the light stays lit. But that's exactly what can happen to nerves in the brain and nervous system when pain signals are turned on.

PAIN AS AN ALTERED STATE

The nervous system, it turns out, is not just a static conduit for relaying signals—it is an actively changing participant in the pain process. While pain generally starts with a physical cause, when it persists it can cause peripheral nerve fibers at the site of the injury to become more sensitive so that even the slightest touch can feel excruciating, a condition known as allodynia.

Unrelenting pain can eventually cause peripheral nerves to communicate their "touchiness" to other nerves along the pain pathway in a noxious process known as sensitization. Essentially, the nervous system in this situation is being "trained" to feel pain. Increasingly, scientists realize that nerves can actually change and grow in new ways that can make pain even more intense, persistent, and widespread. As a result, you can start feeling new pain in places that have nothing to do with the original injury itself, known as referred pain. (Heart attacks, for example, often cause referred pain in an arm or the jaw). Pain can also seep throughout the body, a phenomenon known as radiating pain.

This hellish cascade of pain not only serves no useful biological function, it crosses the line into a harmful condition in which normally healthy processes career out of control. "The idea that pain itself can become a disease of the nervous system has just crystallized in recent years," says Dr. Fine of the University of Utah. "It's becoming clear that while treating an underlying disease or condition is vitally important, it's also important to treat the pain itself, because if you don't, pain is likely to get worse."

Relief ▸**TIP**

Preemptive analgesia, patients not only get a knock-you-out general anesthetic before an operation, but a local painkiller at the site of the incision or perhaps a spinal cord injection to numb the body from the waist down, depending on the procedure. Some studies suggest patients given extra medication have less pain after the operation, fewer complications, and shorter hospital stays.

PEERING AT PAIN

The largely invisible reality that people can experience pain despite the lack of an obvious cause has been substantially illuminated in recent years with brain imaging technologies that allow researchers to watch the brain in action. Studies using magnetic resonance imaging (MRI) and positron emission tomography (PET) scans have clearly shown activity in parts of the brain associated with pain even in cases where there was no physical injury.

HOW PAIN CAN PROGRESS

Think of the way you react when pain first strikes. You flinch, you cringe, you guard the injury by tightening your muscles or perhaps adjusting your posture. These are normal reactions and may not produce any lasting harm in the short term, but over time they can kick off a process that leads to more pain. For example, tightening your neck and shoulder muscles in response to a migraine headache may cause pain in those areas that persists after the headache is gone. Or limping because you have arthritis in your hip may change your posture in ways that cause agony in your lower back.

Chronic pain from such physical de-conditioning and other causes is often matched by an equally important emotional de-conditioning in the form of negative feelings such as demoralization, depression, and anxiety—all of which can be aggravated by pain-related loss of sleep. This deconditioning can become a vicious circle. "Pain can cause a decay of the human spirit that some research suggests may actually predispose you to lower thresholds for musculoskeletal pain," says Fine.

As pain persists, it can cause changes or damage to the nervous system itself, a concept known as plasticity, which scientists are only beginning to understand. In addition to nerve cells becoming hypersensitive, unremitting pain appears able to:

■ Make damaged nerve fibers fire spontaneously and intensely, often producing a burning sensation similar to an electric shock.

■ Reorganize connections between nerve fibers so new connections are formed to produce pain that otherwise wouldn't have existed.

■ Change the chemistry of pain processing so that endorphins are prevented from dialing back the volume on pain, perhaps due to a genetic deficiency.

Understanding that such changes take place—and gaining insights into how they work—is a major advance in pain medicine that points the way to potential new treatments. "Things are evolving very quickly," says Fine. Meanwhile, existing therapies can go a long way toward providing relief.

THE MYSTERIES OF PHANTOM PAIN

Doctors have long puzzled over why up to half of people whose limbs have been amputated due to wounds, accidents, or disease continue feeling pain in the missing body part. The pain is unique to each person. Although the exact mechanism is still not clear, it's possible that the brain contains an internal blueprint of the body—a reason why children born without limbs can experience phantom pain as readily as people whose limbs are removed. But pain may also occur as the brain compensates for the confusing loss of signals from the missing part by forming new connections that create false sensations. Many amputees develop a "trigger zone," a sensitive area of the body that mimics signals for the missing limb. A breeze blowing against the amputee's face, for example, may register as a touch on his phantom body part.

DO KIDS REMEMBER PAIN?

Pain in children has often been disregarded because it's assumed kids don't recall their pain, so it does no lasting harm. However, recent research has called this view into question by suggesting that unpleasant sensations such as needle sticks alter the pain-processing wiring in developing brains. In one of the most significant studies, boys who were circumcised (a procedure usually done without anesthetic) reacted more strongly than uncircumcised boys to a routine vaccination at age 4 to 6 months. This suggests that, although infants may not consciously remember a given encounter with pain, the sensations register at the biological level and may have an impact on pain perception later in life.

2

MAINSTREAM MEDICINE

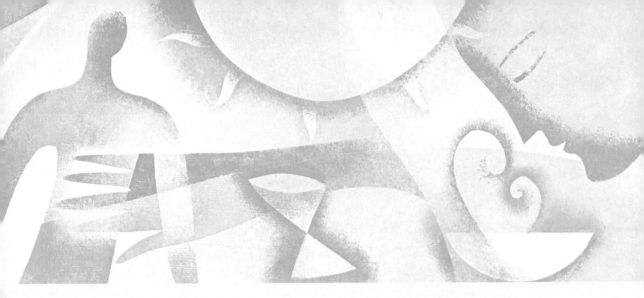

The development of anesthetics and pain-relieving drugs in the mid-1800s revolutionized the practice of medicine. Surgeries that would have been—and often were—barbaric before the use of ether in the operating room could now save lives. Even the manufacture of pain- and inflammation-relieving aspirin didn't come until the turn of the 20th century. Now—thanks to burgeoning scientific research—doctors can offer patients a battery of options for relieving pain with many more possibilities on the horizon.

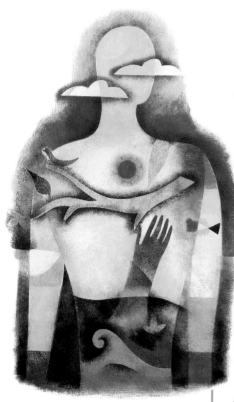

For most of history, there wasn't much that doctors, surgeons, dentists, or barbers—all considered roughly the same profession—could do to stop pain. Then, in the 19th century, a series of discoveries paved the way for modern pain medicine—perhaps the most important medical advances of all time.

Until doctors figured out a way to numb the nervous system's pain pathways, medicine, particularly surgery, was barbaric. A doctor was said to come into the operating room with two bottles of whiskey—one for the patient and the other for himself—to cope with the patient's screaming. People with chronic pain were largely left to suffer.

The Advent of Pain Medicine

What changed medicine was the development of pain-relieving drugs and anesthetics based on natural substances: nitrous oxide (laughing gas); chloroform, a gas that rendered people unconscious; and ether, a safer (though highly flammable) knockout gas that became the first widely used general anesthesia. Just as important have been medicines from plant sources like the opium poppy, the coca leaf, and willow bark—from which we still get the pain-relieving drugs morphine, procaine (Novocain), and aspirin.

Today, patients and doctors have a wide range of medical treatments available for mediating pain, including:

- Tried-and-true drugs such as morphine that have been used for more than a century
- New forms of narcotic medications, called opiods, that provide choices in strength and length of action
- A new class of anti-inflammatory drugs that relieve pain just like their older cousins but with fewer of the most significant side effects
- Combination drugs that mix and match different drugs' pain-relieving powers and potential side effects to maximum advantage

- Medicines that are usually prescribed for other conditions, such as depression, but also fight pain
- A variety of ways to administer drugs, including portable pump systems that patients can control themselves
- Spinal cord stimulators
- Surgery blocks
- Surgeries to treat painful underlying conditions

Assessing the Agony

Given the variety of today's options, where should you and your doctor start when deciding on a pain treatment? A doctor can't suggest a course of action until he or she knows how much you're suffering. Your pain may be perfectly obvious to you, but it won't necessarily be clear to your physician.

"Pain is completely subjective," says Melvin C. Gitlin, M.D., professor and chairman of the department of anesthesiology at Tulane University School of Medicine, director of the Pain

ANESTHESIA'S "AHA" MOMENTS

A number of people share credit for the discovery of anesthesia in the 19th century, even though the basic ingredients had been available for years.

In fact, ether and nitrous oxide were scientifically established as painkillers only after laughing gas parties and "ether frolics," in which the then-unregulated gases were used for social entertainment, became the rage in the mid-1800s.

At one such party, a Georgia doctor named Crawford Long noticed that after inhaling the gas, partygoers didn't feel pain when they bumped into things. Sharing this observation, one of Long's friends allowed the doctor to remove two small tumors from his neck in 1842, using ether successfully to quell the pain. But because his discovery wasn't published for years, Long's pioneering operation went largely unnoticed.

A few years later, however, in a famous demonstration in the operating theater at Massachusetts General Hospital, a dentist named William Morton (who had designed ether inhalers for use on his patients) anesthetized a patient for a jaw-tumor operation before an intent audience of skeptical doctors. (A well-known surgeon, Dr. John C. Warren, performed the actual operation.) When the patient awoke feeling no pain, the audience was electrified, and word spread around the world that, as one London newspaper put it, "We have conquered pain." The operating room, later known as the Ether Dome, is today a museum.

THE INITIAL VISIT: WHAT TO EXPECT

Pain is the number one reason people see doctors, but complaining that you hurt is just a starting point, according to Melvin Gitlin, M.D., of the American Academy of Pain Medicine. To help steer your treatment—both for pain and its underlying cause—your doctor will go through a number of steps to learn more about your problem, including:

Taking a history

Often accomplished by a questionnaire and a conversation, your history tells your doctor:

- What health problems you've experienced
- How your pain behaves
- Whether illnesses in members of your family put you at risk for certain painful conditions
- What medications you're currently taking (which can have a bearing on treatment options)

Performing a physical exam

Your doctor will want to make a direct observation of your body, which may involve some poking and prodding to establish where the pain is located and what affects it.

Reviewing prior tests

If you've been to other doctors for your problem, your new physician will want to look over results from all previous tests before deciding on any new ones you might need—or making a better diagnosis on the basis of what's been learned already.

Management Center at Tulane's Health Sciences Center, and 2003 president of the American Academy of Pain Medicine. "You can't measure it with a blood test or see it under a microscope. For example, if I look at an X ray of a broken leg, I can guess that a person is hurting, but one person may experience the pain as severe and another person may experience it as moderate."

Fortunately, there are a number of ways for your doctor to learn more about how you're feeling. Quantifying and describing pain not only helps guide treatment choices at the outset, says Gitlin, it establishes a benchmark for how effectively the therapy is working and provides the basis for future decisions.

TELLING THE TORTURE TALE

Every pain has a story, and it's up to you to convey it to your doctor. Describing your pain may not be as easy as it sounds. You may wonder why saying "it hurts" isn't enough. But pain assessments can reveal important details about your pain that help doctors get a better picture of what's happening. These include:

- Where the pain is located
- When it started
- When it tends to get worse
- What seems to make it better
- How long flare-ups usually last
- How intensely you feel pain physically
- How it affects you psychologically
- How the quality of the pain makes it different from other pains

Many of these points are fairly simple to address—when and where pain tends to occur, for example. But conveying the finer points of intensity, quality, and psychological impact may require the use of assessment tools.

The first step is often to quantify how badly you hurt, which can be done with a number of methods, including:

Visual Analog Scales

One of the simplest pain measures, the visual analog scale, consists of a single horizontal line (typically about 4 inches wide) with two extremes of pain experience on opposite ends—"no pain" on one side and "worst pain imaginable" (or words to that effect) on the other. You simply place a mark on the line to indicate where you feel your pain falls on the continuum—perhaps with the help of a ruler-like device with a sliding indicator line. The test is fast, easy, and reliable, though some people find it a bit abstract, due to the blank scale's lack of marks or numbers. It looks like this:

No Pain   Worst Pain Imaginable

Numbered Scales

Numerical rating scales are similar to visual analog scales except numbers are placed along the line that help you put a value on your pain. Typically, the numbers run from 0 on the "no pain" side to 10 on the "worst pain" side, though there are also scales that run from 0 to 100. Assigning a number to pain helps some people communicate their experience more clearly. But needing to choose specific points along the scale makes it less sensitive than visual analog scales in picking up subtle degrees of difference between points. A typical numbered scale looks like this:

0   1   2   3   4   5   6   7   8   9   10

No Pain   Worst Pain Imaginable

Verbal Scales

Verbal rating scales use the same idea of a one-extreme-to-the-other line, but mark the line with words that describe how intense your pain may be. You choose the word that best describes what you feel. Verbal scales share the simplicity of numbered and visual scales, but tend to limit your choices even more—especially because people usually gravitate to the even more limited number of descriptive words in the middle of the scale. A typical example might look like this:

No pain   Annoying   Uncomfortable   Dreadful   Horrible   Agonizing

PREPARING FOR A PAIN ASSESSMENT

Your doctor should have a lot of questions for you about your pain. While you may prefer to think about something else, considering your answers ahead of time can help ease the flow of conversation and allow for a more comprehensive discussion with your physician. If it helps, go over potential questions with a trusted friend or family member who can accompany you to the assessment. If you find it difficult to speak or concentrate, that person can answer for you. In addition to the qualities of the pain itself, consider whether (or how) your pain:

✱ Disrupts your sleep

✱ Changes your appetite

✱ Affects your mood

✱ Keeps you from doing things you'd like to do

✱ Limits your mobility

✱ Restricts your social life

✱ Affects your relationships

THE POWER OF OBSERVATION

While not as reliable as patient self-reporting, your doctor will also try to gauge your pain with his own eyes—partly by watching how you behave. While you shouldn't "act to the camera" of your doctor's gaze—some data suggests that doctors don't take patients as seriously if they are too emotional or agitated—you also shouldn't try to be stoic to a physician who can read valuable clues in your:

✱ Facial expressions such as grimaces or flinches

✱ Posture

✱ "Guarding" behavior in which you try to protect the pained site from further discomfort

Other Approaches

Pain questionnaires may include a variety of these scales—and some others besides. For example, people who are already being treated for pain may be evaluated with a scale showing how well pain is being relieved, with words like "No relief of pain" on one side and "Complete relief of pain" on the other. Other scales use a series of circles containing "smiley faces," which become progressively less smiley and more agonized to indicate points along the pain continuum—an approach that's particularly useful with children who may have trouble understanding verbal or numerical concepts.

THE MCGILL PAIN QUESTIONNAIRE

Pain scales have limits: They don't address the quality of pain, but instead treat all types of pain as if they were a single experience that simply gets more or less intense. The pains of a heart attack, a toothache, an electrical burn, and neuropathy from diabetes all feel different. It's just as important to explain what kind of pain you're experiencing as it is to nail down its intensity.

One pain assessment tool that captures how pain feels is the McGill Pain Questionnaire, a kind of extended verbal scale that lets respondents choose from a range of words to describe their pain. The words themselves come from patients' own accounts of pain in studies, and the list has been expanded over the years to provide a remarkably comprehensive catalog of pain language. Studies find that people suffering from the same condition tend to be surprisingly consistent in the words they choose to describe pain—"gnawing" and "aching" for arthritis, for example. That's important because it means the way you describe your pain provides clues about what may be causing it. What's more, researchers have found that the words on the test can be accurately scored to reflect pain's intensity as well. "The McGill Pain Questionnaire is a time-honored test, and one of the most commonly used," says Gitlin of the American Academy of Pain Medicine. "It's my personal favorite."

THE PARLANCE OF PAIN

According to the developers of the McGill Pain Questionnaire (one of whom, Ronald Melzak, also helped develop the gate control theory), words for pain can be grouped into three distinct categories, all of which help reveal the nature of pain for the sufferer:

PAIN QUALITY	WHAT IT MEANS	VERBAL DESCRIPTION
Sensory	How pain feels physically	Throbbing, pounding, shooting, stabbing, sharp, pinching, pressing, crushing, tugging, wrenching, burning, scalding, tingling, smarting, stinging, dull, sore, aching, tender, taut, splitting
Affective	How pain feels emotionally	Tiring, exhausting, sickening, suffocating, frightful, terrifying, punishing, grueling, cruel, wretched, blinding
Evaluative	How you judge the experience of pain	Annoying, troublesome, miserable, intense, unbearable

KEEPING A PAIN DIARY

Pain assessments measure your pain at the moment you take them. The perspective you gain by keeping track of your pain over time can help fill in the details of your pain history (such as when pain occurs and what makes it better or worse). One way to do it is to keep a pain diary or journal, rating your pain on a simple scale perhaps three times a day—in the morning, at lunch and at bedtime—or anytime pain flares up. (See page 42 for a sample form.) Keeping a log can reveal pain patterns that may go unnoticed if you were to rely entirely on memory.

The more detailed your records, the more helpful they'll be. Among the details that are worth noting:

- What you were doing when you rated your pain
- Any medications you've taken—and when
- Flare-ups that seem to strike at unexpected times (and what you were doing then as well)
- Your mood, to get a sense of the interplay between your emotions and your pain
- How well you sleep—and how much

By seeing how your pain scores may change over time, writing a daily account of your pain can foster an encouraging sense of progress even if it feels like you're struggling from day to day. Bonus: Simply writing down an account of your pain and your feelings can help provide emotional release and a sense of support—even if no one else reads your diary.

Daily Pain Diary

Date: _____

Time	Intensity of pain from 0 (none) to 10 (worst ever)	Description of pain	What you were doing	Medication taken type/amount	Nondrug techniques tried	Comments (mood, other symptoms, sleep quality)
Midnight						
1 A.M.						
2 A.M.						
3 A.M.						
4 A.M.						
5 A.M.						
6 A.M.						
7 A.M.						
8 A.M.						
9 A.M.						
10 A.M.						
11 A.M.						
Noon						
1 P.M.						
2 P.M.						
3 P.M.						
4 P.M.						
5 P.M.						
6 P.M.						
7 P.M.						
8 P.M.						
9 P.M.						
10 P.M.						
11 P.M.						

Managing Pain with Medication

With more than 20 painkilling medications available from one prescription class alone (nonsteroidal anti-inflammatory drugs, or NSAIDs), there's no shortage of drugs that can help ease your discomfort. The challenge, in fact, is to find the drug (or combination of drugs) that best balances pain-relieving power with side effects in your specific case. You'll need to work out an approach with your doctor, but the chances are good that your pain can be alleviated.

It's important to realize that, while drugs can be said to have certain general properties, not everyone reacts to medications the same way. "The drugs in a given class are mostly the same, but subtle chemical variations can make a difference in the way your body absorbs it, how quickly it crosses from the blood to the brain, and how it affects other body functions to produce side effects," says Perry Fine, M.D., associate medical director of the University of Utah Pain Management Center. "There's no good way to predict how you'll respond to a certain medication once an assessment determines it's appropriate for you, other than to give it a try." That's why people with chronic pain change their medications an average of three times a year, Fine says.

The takeaway: While it can be frustrating if a medication doesn't cut your pain as much as you'd like, take your dissatisfaction as a sign of progress—knowing what doesn't work moves you one step closer to what does. Your doctor can help you make new choices from the following menu of drug types.

THE WORD ON NSAIDS

Because the body's pain-producing process is largely related to the swelling, redness, heat, and pain of inflammation, controlling one of its root causes—the production of hormone-like prostaglandins—is a key way to ease certain types of pain. The

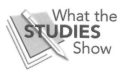

What the STUDIES Show

Do NSAIDs prevent uterine cancer? Preliminary research at the University of Illinois suggests the answer may be yes. In a lab study, malignant cells taken from the lining of the uterus made neighboring healthy cells produce COX-2 enzymes, setting in motion a cascade of reactions that can contribute to tumor growth. Drugs that suppress COX-2 production, such as COX-2 inhibitors and other NSAIDs, are already prescribed to treat colon cancer and precancerous colon polyps. Further study may reveal that they help prevent uterine cancer as well.

main weapons for doing so are nonsteroidal anti-inflammatory drugs, or NSAIDs. Often the first weapons drawn in the battle against pain, NSAIDs are particularly useful for treating pain from arthritis, muscle sprains and strains, headaches, backaches, and neck injuries.

NSAIDs are probably the most familiar pain medications because a number of them are sold over the counter. Aspirin—first marketed as a pain reliever in the late 19th century—is one. So are ibuprofen (marketed under brand names such as Advil, Motrin, and Nuprin), naproxen sodium (Aleve), and ketoprofen (Orudis KT). But there's also an extensive line of more potent prescription NSAIDs such as nabumetone (Relafen), piroxicam (Feldene), and sulindac (Clinoril).

Whatever their names, all NSAIDs block production of pain-causing prostaglandins by suppressing the action of an enzyme called cyclooxygenase (COX). This enzyme comes in two forms, COX-1 and COX-2, and squelching either of them (especially COX-2) stems the tide of prostaglandins.

Just one hitch: As noted in chapter 1, prostaglandins play a lot of important roles in the body, and limiting their function across the board creates some drawbacks. Particularly pertinent: The COX-1 enzyme also produces "good" prostaglandins that help protect the lining of the gastrointestinal tract from caustic digestive juices. Taking it out of action leaves the stomach and GI tract vulnerable to significant problems, including ulcers, bleeding, and—paradoxically—pain.

SORTING OUT NSAIDs

Although there are many different NSAIDs, researchers sort them into four basic groups:

CATEGORY	EXAMPLE	OFTEN USED FOR
Low potency, short acting	Ibuprofen (Advil, Motrin, Nuprin)	Acute pain, rheumatoid arthritis
High potency, short acting	Diclofenac (Voltaren)	Rheumatoid arthritis, osteoarthritis
Intermediate potency, intermediate acting	Naproxen (Anaprox DS, Naprelan, Naprosyn)	Migraines, myofascial pain, menstrual pain
High potency, long acting	Piroxicam (Feldene)	Multiple forms of arthritis, cancer, myofascial pain

Should you use NSAIDs? Keep in mind that not everyone who takes an NSAID will react to it the same way. If you can't tolerate one drug in this class, another may work better. What's more, significant side effects often don't show up unless you use NSAIDs regularly—perhaps for months or even years. Occasional use (especially in low doses) is generally safe. Work with your doctor to make the best choice—and speak up if your gut starts giving you grief.

COX-2 INHIBITORS: BEST OF BOTH WORLDS?

It's not often that a new type of pain medicine is hailed as a breakthrough, but that's what happened in the late 1990s, when a new class of painkillers came on the market in the form of the drugs celecoxib (Celebrex) and rofecoxib (Vioxx). Called COX-2 inhibitors, these drugs are NSAIDs that target only the COX-2 enzyme while leaving the gut-protecting COX-1 enzyme alone. (Scientists didn't realize there were two COX enzymes until the early 1990s.) Result: COX-2 inhibitors quell pain just as well as—though not better than—standard NSAIDs, while avoiding the older drugs' most noxious side effects.

With such a wonderful résumé, you'd think COX-2s would make other NSAIDs obsolete. But while a great deal of excitement still surrounds COX-2s (as early as 1999, a third of arthritis patients had prescriptions for them), a second glance produces a more balanced picture.

First, like most drugs that are new (i.e., still under patent), COX-2s cost more than their older cousins. "Unless gastrointestinal side effects are already an issue for you, there's no sense writing a prescription for an appreciably more expensive drug when something you can buy off the shelf at the corner pharmacy may work just as well," says Fine. Beyond that, studies suggest that COX-2 inhibitors may boost your risk of blood clots and, potentially, cardiovascular problems. What's more, while they have fewer gastrointestinal side effects than other NSAIDs, COX-2s still cause gut trouble for some people.

Bottom line: COX-2s are a valuable addition to the painkilling arsenal, but they're not risk-free and their long-term

THE NEWEST COX-2

In mid-2002, the Food and Drug Administration approved a third COX-2 drug. Called valdecoxib (Bextra), it's similar to the two existing COX-2s and is primarily meant to treat osteoarthritis, rheumatoid arthritis, and menstrual pain and cramping but not acute pain. Valdecoxib does an even better job of selectively targeting the COX-2 enzyme than other drugs in this class, which may make it a good choice for people most at risk of gastrointestinal bleeding from NSAIDs, but it also appears in studies to further boost heart risks from blood clotting.

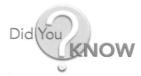

safety isn't as well established as that of older NSAIDs. You may be a candidate for COX-2s if you have ulcers, haven't been able to tolerate other NSAIDs, or are older than 65, when bleeding and other side effects from NSAIDs are more likely.

ACETAMINOPHEN: THE NON-NSAID

Until acetaminophen (Tylenol, Panadol) hit the market around 1960, aspirin was the only over-the-counter pain reliever available—a position it had held for more than half a century. Still often mentioned in the same breath as aspirin and other NSAIDs, acetaminophen is the odd man out because it's not an NSAID at all. That's because it doesn't affect prostaglandins and thus does nothing to fight inflammation. Yet it relieves certain types of pain just as well as NSAIDs do. For example, it's a good first option for pain such as osteoarthritis, which generally doesn't involve inflammation. Researchers aren't entirely sure how acetaminophen eases pain, but it appears to work directly on the central nervous system.

Because it doesn't suppress prostaglandins (or the enzymes that trigger them), acetaminophen is far gentler on the stomach and gastrointestinal tract than NSAIDs. It also tends to interact well with other medications, so it's sometimes used to give stronger medicines like narcotics an added pain-relieving boost. Aside from the fact that it's of limited benefit for inflammatory pain like rheumatoid arthritis, acetaminophen has other drawbacks. The main concern is that high doses or regular use over an extended period of time (typically years) can increase your risk of liver or kidney damage. Alcohol boosts this risk considerably: Even casual users can suffer serious liver problems if they have as few as three drinks a day while on acetaminophen. Taking acetaminophen with food helps reduce these risks, but you're best off avoiding alcohol entirely while using the drug, and sticking to doses well below the recommended daily maximum of 4,000 mg, particularly if you take other medications that contain acetaminophen.

CORTICOSTEROIDS: AN ANTI-INFLAMMATORY OPTION

Saying NSAIDs are "nonsteroidal" is a way of making clear they don't fall into this next category of painkiller. Corticosteroids (sometimes just called "steroids") are synthetic drugs that chemically resemble natural hormones in the body. Among their effects: They reduce inflammation and swelling even better than NSAIDs, making them potent painkillers, especially for inflammatory pain from cancer, compressed nerves, and musculoskeletal disorders like rheumatoid arthritis. In fact, when they were first introduced in the 1950s, they were hailed as a breakthrough treatment for rheumatoid arthritis patients, who often found that just a few days on these drugs could significantly improve mobility.

Unfortunately, having powerful pain-relieving effects means corticosteroids have potent side effects as well. Today, corticosteroids are seldom prescribed for more than several weeks at a time, to prevent problems such as ulcers, marked weight gain (which can lead to high blood pressure), calcium loss that can cause osteoporosis, menstrual irregularities, and other effects ranging from mood changes to fatty bulges on the back.

Still, corticosteroids are often used as a fallback treatment that can provide welcome relief, especially for people with severe joint or cancer pain. To minimize steroids' side effects, doctors often inject them directly into a joint or other site of pain to contain their action to a specific area. (Pills send drugs coursing through the entire body.) Fortunately, if side effects become intolerable, they'll usually disappear once you stop taking the drug.

OPIOIDS: THE POWERHOUSE PAINKILLERS

Few drugs stir up more controversy than opioids, natural and synthetic narcotics. But there's one thing everybody agrees on: They're the most potent pain relievers available, and are the mainstays of pain management.

Opioids get their name from the opium poppy, which has been a source of folk and traditional remedies (and yes, abuse) for centuries. Some of the best-known opioids are natural forms such as morphine and codeine, but by isolating and tinkering with the more than 20 compounds in opium, scientists have come up with a variety of synthetic siblings. Opioid drugs differ from each other in how strong they are, how quickly they take effect, and how long they last, but all essentially do the same thing—act like an "off" switch for pain.

Think of neurons (nerve cells) as rooftop TV antennas that receive pain signals, but can't provide a clear pain picture when

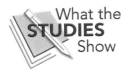

What the STUDIES Show

In one recent study that used national databases to track trends with several popular opioid medications (including morphine and oxycodone), researchers found that during a six-year period, overall abuse went down. The kicker: During the same period, the number of prescriptions for the drugs increased several times over— evidence that more legitimate drug use doesn't produce more addiction.

birds perch on their wires. Opioids are like flocks of birds that gather on your pain antennae, turning savage signals to a soothing hiss. On cells, special "perches" for opioids are called receptors, and they're found throughout the body, not just on nerve cells—one reason opioids can cause a variety of side effects. Your "perches" may be somewhat different than your neighbor's, so some birds—that is, medications—may find it easier to perch with you than others. Some will tend to flutter off after a short time and some will linger longer. But whatever your pain, there's probably an opioid that can help.

Doctors classify opioids in various ways, but the drugs basically break down into two categories:

Weak opioids. These drugs aren't necessarily feeble—they're just not as potent as strong opioids and are typically used for mild to moderate pain. When combined, nonsteroidal and opioid drugs appear to boost each other's potency, and weak opioids such as codeine and hydrocodone are often mixed with acetaminophen and aspirin to get more pain-relieving power with less opioid medication—and fewer narcotic side effects.

Strong opioids. Morphine, the granddaddy of narcotics (and still the gold standard), is among the most widely prescribed strong opioids, which also include methadone, fentanyl, hydromorphone and oxycodone. Strong opioids are generally reserved for severe pain.

One of the most common side effects of opioid use is drowsiness, though sedation varies depending on the drug you're taking and the dose. Drowsiness isn't necessarily bad: If the torment of pain has been wrecking your sleep, you may count drowsiness as a plus. In some cases, drowsiness that you think comes from the drug is actually sleep debt, which will disappear after a night or two of decent rest. Other common side effects include constipation due to opioids' tendency to slow bowel movement, really the number one problem for patients; nausea and vomiting; loss of appetite; swelling, itching, low testosterone, and slowing of your breathing—potentially serious, but not likely to be a problem if you take the right dose. All these side effects often slack off or even disappear after a few weeks of taking the medication, but if problems persist, talk to your doctor about adjusting the dose or switching to a new drug.

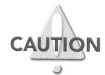

CAUTION

If you're being treated for chronic pain, avoid using meperidine (Demerol), an opioid popular for easing acute pain after surgeries. The reason: During metabolism, the drug creates byproducts that have been linked to muscle spasms, mental confusion, and seizures—effects that can outlast the medication's pain-relieving benefits and be intensified by the presence of other medications.

DO OPIOIDS CAUSE ADDICTION?

If the word "narcotics" makes you think of stupefied street addicts, gang wars, and police sirens, you're not alone. About half of patients who have taken opioid painkillers say they're concerned about becoming addicted, according to a survey from the American Academy of Pain Medicine and the American Pain Society. Many other patients and doctors simply avoid opioids, fearing the drugs will either become habit-forming or lead to trouble with the law.

There's reason for concern. In many states, doctors can be prosecuted for overprescribing narcotics—and in some well-publicized cases, physicians have been charged as dealers. Recently, drug abusers have discovered they can get a huge "rush" by crushing and snorting OxyContin, a sustained-release formulation of the opioid oxycodone. In one year alone, emergency room reports involving oxycodone jumped 68 percent, and there have been hundreds of overdose deaths. OxyContin incidents are still only 2 percent of those associated with heroin, cocaine, alcohol, and other drugs.

But while these issues get all the press, pain management experts say the addiction danger is vastly overstated. "The idea that you'll become addicted using opioids for pain is not borne out by doctors' own experience, and it's not supported by the medical literature," says Melvin Gitlin, M.D., 2003 president of the American Academy of Pain Medicine (AAPM). Some research suggests that less than 5 percent of people who regularly take opioids for pain become addicted. (Other estimates are below 1 percent.) In a joint position paper, the AAPM and the American Pain Society say groundless fears cause many people to suffer needlessly "despite the ready availability of safe and effective treatments."

A key to clearing up this confusion is to understand the difference between tolerance, dependence, and addiction—terms with very different meanings that are often used interchangeably.

Tolerance: The same amount of drug becomes less effective over time as your body adjusts to it, so you have to bump up the dose. To some extent, tolerance is good: It's the reason opioid side effects level off soon after you start. Fortunately, tolerance of opioids' painkilling power tapers off much more slowly than side effects. Recent research suggests it's not as big a problem as previously thought. "In most cases, it turns out people need more drugs because their disease has gotten worse, not because the medication is less effective," says Gitlin.

Dependence: Your body becomes accustomed to a drug and you'll suffer withdrawal symptoms, such as anxiety, sweating, or sleep loss, if you suddenly stop taking it. Dependence is normal when you're repeatedly exposed to a drug and isn't necessarily harmful—if it were, the caffeine you crave in your morning coffee would be outlawed. You can sidestep withdrawal problems by decreasing your dosage gradually.

Addiction: A psychological problem in which you become fixated on using a drug not to ease pain and make your health better, but to get high. Few patients taking opioids for pain feel compelled to use more than they need to ease their suffering (often because of side effects), and addiction is rare in pain management. For example, in two studies of opioid use for back pain—at Harvard University and the San Francisco Spine Institute—a total of 99 patients got narcotics, but only one showed signs of abusing them.

DOUBLE-IDENTITY DRUGS

Like comic book characters whose everyday identities disguise surprising powers, a number of drugs normally considered treatments for problems like depression, anxiety, and seizures have also been found to be super pain fighters. Often lumped together in a category called adjuvant medications, these drugs include:

Tricyclic antidepressants. These blues battlers work by boosting levels of two chemicals—serotonin and norepineph-rine—that chase away clouds of gloom in the brain but also block pain signals as they move up the spinal cord. Tricyclics are particularly good at relieving sharp, shooting, or burning pain from damaged or compressed nerves, and are often used for people with diabetes, cancer, fibromyalgia, or spinal cord injuries. Side effects include dry mouth, weight gain, low blood

COMMONLY USED OPIOIDS

TYPE	NAME	DELIVERY	COMMENTS
Weak	Codeine	Tablet, liquid	Often mixed with aspirin or acetaminophen. Usually taken every 4 hours.
	Hydrocodone	Tablet	Usually mixed with aspirin or acetaminophen. Slightly stronger than codeine.
	Propoxyphene	Tablet	Weakest of the opioids. Most effective when mixed with aspirin every 4 to 6 hours.
Strong	Fentanyl	Skin patch	Extremely potent, but patch eases it slowly into the body over two or three days for steady relief.
	Hydromorphone	Tablet, injection, suppository	Common alternative to morphine, but about 7 times more potent and usually faster-acting.
	Levorphanol	Tablet, injection	Five times more potent than morphine (orally), and longer-lasting.
	Methadone	Tablet, injection	Takes up to 3 or 4 days to clear the body, so side effects may be long-lasting. Proper dosing trickier than with most opioids.
	Morphine	Tablet, liquid, injection, suppository	Standard by which other opioids are measured. Available in a variety of concentrations and formulations, some of which are controlled release.
	Oxycodone	Tablet	Often used with aspirin or acetaminophen for moderate pain, or by itself for stronger pain.

pressure, sedation (they're often taken before bed), and urinary retention, but with a range of tricyclics available, there's probably one that you'd find tolerable.

Anticonvulsants. No drugs are specifically made to battle the haywire sparking of nerves known as neuropathy—and pain from the condition isn't easily relieved with opioids or other painkillers. That makes drugs that prevent seizures a godsend. By controlling the abnormal firing of nerves that causes problems like convulsions, anticonvulsants also quiet the erratic signals that bring on stabs of neuropathic pain. Anticonvulsants also block sodium channels (see below). Side effects include dizziness, drowsiness, nausea, constipation, and, more rarely, heart, blood, and liver problems, though most people find the drugs easy to tolerate.

Sodium channel blockers. When all else fails, some doctors bring in drugs such as sodium channel blockers that usually are prescribed to control abnormal electrical rhythms in the heart. Because pain is also an electrical process, these drugs can help quell pain-producing nerve impulses as well. Sodium channel blockers should be used with caution, however, to make sure the heart keeps beating properly, and doctors often prescribe them only in low doses in conjunction with other pain medications.

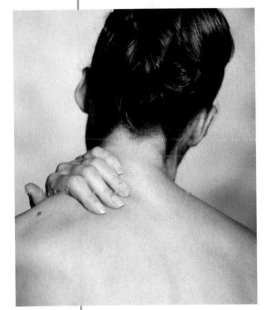

RUBBING OUT PAIN

For most drugs to do their magic, you have to get them inside the body, but some medications for pain work from the outside—in the form of creams and gels that you rub on your skin.

Among these are capsaicin, a medication made from chili peppers, available over the counter in products such as Zostrix. You rub capsaicin on your skin several times a day, which stimulates the release of substance P, a protein that helps nerves pass pain signals along. That sounds bad—and for a time, in fact, capsaicin causes a burning irritation. But if you keep treatment up for a week or two, the constant stimulation uses up substance P at the site, subduing pain (along with the peppery irritation). Capsaicin works best against pain near the surface of the skin, such as arthritis in the fingers, knees, and elbows; nerve pain that follows a bout with shingles;

nerve pain from diabetes; and pain from surgical scars.

Other topical treatments include over-the-counter ointments such as Ben-Gay and Icy Hot, which provide relief by using heat or cold sensations to load nerves with competing signals, masking pain. Though they're of limited use for severe, chronic pain, these products can help soothe aching muscles.

OTHER OPTIONS

Some medications for pain don't fit neatly into other drug categories but may nevertheless provide significant relief for some people. Among them:

Tramadol. Marketed under the brand name Ultram, this drug is a very weak narcotic (not considered a controlled substance by the DEA) that latches onto opioid receptors on cells. Like a tricyclic antidepressant, it boosts levels of serotonin and norepinephrine. The fact that it works in both ways makes it an effective pain reliever that's about as potent as codeine. Many doctors prescribe it as an intermediate step between less powerful NSAIDs and more potent narcotics. Because it binds weakly to opioid receptors, tramadol has many of the same side effects as narcotics, such as sedation, nausea, and constipation, and it may have a higher risk of seizures.

Botox. It's most famous as a wrinkle remover, but botulinum toxin—botox for short—has been approved for years to treat conditions such as strabismus (wandering eye). More recently, doctors have successfully used it to treat no fewer than 25 problems related to muscle spasms, many of which produce pain. One of the world's most potent toxins, botox seems an improbable medicine. But when injected into isolated areas of the body, its poisonous effects are limited to blocking nerve signals to specific muscles, making them relax. Though not well studied, preliminary research suggests it may also be helpful for migraine headaches and some types of back pain. In one study, botox injections eliminated recurring headaches in more than half of patients and halved the number of headaches for another 35 percent. A small study at the Uniformed Services University in Bethesda, Maryland, found botox cut back pain by at least half in 78 percent of people who got it. It's also been used to ease painful muscle spasms in stroke victims and to relieve writer's cramp.

People usually stop using drugs not because they're ineffective or addictive, but because side effects seem worse than the pain the products are supposed to relieve. While you almost always have options for new treatments, you can also relieve common side effects with simple steps. Here's what to do in case of…

SIDE EFFECT	REMEDIES
Drowsiness	■ Wait a few days and take pleasure in sleeping better: Sedation often eases soon after starting a new drug. ■ Consider whether your pain medication is really at fault. Other drugs (antihistamines, for example) can also make you groggy. ■ Ask your doctor to prescribe smaller amounts that you take more often to soften each dose's "oomph." Or cut the dose across the board: That can sometimes reduce drowsiness while not substantially cutting pain protection. ■ Consult your doctor if the drug isn't providing enough relief: It you're still in pain, that may be what's wearing you out, not the drug.
Constipation	■ Drink more water. You should down at least eight cups of water a day—a standard recommendation that most people nevertheless don't follow. ■ Eat high-fiber foods such as raw fruits, vegetables, and whole-grain breads and cereals, which add bulk and help stools absorb water. Another option: Be a high-fiber bran fanatic. Keep a bran-filled shaker on the table so you can dash it on foods. ■ Have your physician recommend a stool softener and suggest a dose. ■ Try to exercise as much as you're able: Physical activity helps keep the bowels in motion. ■ Try to avoid laxatives or bowel stimulants that your gut will become dependent on.
Nausea and vomiting	■ Ask your doctor about taking over-the-counter motion sickness drugs like meclizine and dimenhydrinate or getting a prescription anti-nausea medication. ■ If nausea mostly bothers you when walking around, lie down for an hour or so after taking your medication. ■ Check if other drugs you're taking may be causing your discomfort, and talk to your doctor about adjusting the dose of the likeliest culprit.
Stomach irritation	■ Take your medicine with a glass of water or with food. ■ If you're using NSAIDs, ask your doctor if you can take occasional days off to give your gut time to mend between doses. If your pain won't allow a break, consider switching to acetaminophen or a COX-2 drug. ■ If you're on aspirin, try enteric-coated brands like Ecotrin, which encase the medication so it doesn't dissolve until it passes through the stomach into the small intestine, where it's less likely to cause irritation. Downside: Pain relief is delayed as well. ■ Avoid alcohol or keep drinks to a daily maximum of three: Heavier imbibing makes stomach irritation more likely. ■ Take medications to control reflux and acid production

Your Pain Medication Plan

With so many possible choices, deciding which drugs to take may seem a daunting challenge for you and your doctor. But while each case is different and you'll probably need to go through some trial and error, doctors tend to follow well-established general guidelines when prescribing pain medications.

The process usually begins with a pain assessment like the McGill Pain Questionnaire, both to get a sense of how punishing your pain is and clues about where it comes from (if that's not already known). Next, your doctor will probably work with you to establish goals for your treatment, putting priority on steps that will make pain management progressively easier.

In many cases, the first objective is to relieve nighttime pain so you can get a good night's sleep. If you're well rested, you'll be significantly better able to cope with—and manage—pain during the day.

The next step is often to control pain that occurs when you're awake during the day but not moving around—what's often called resting pain. When resting pain has been eased, you can more effectively battle pain when your body's in motion.

The third goal is generally to relieve pain that may hinder movement that's critical to your quality of life—whether it's getting out of bed, taking a bath, or going back to work.

With your condition and goals established, it's time to come up with the specifics of your treatment, following these guidelines:

- **Start low.** Whether you're taking an NSAID, opioid, or adjuvant medication, expect your doctor to start you on the lowest dose that it's reasonable to expect will ease your pain. This keeps side effects to a minimum and gives you an idea how well you respond to the drug.
- **Look to history.** Your doctor's choice of medication depends first on your condition and medical history. For example, if you have a history of kidney disease or stomach ulcers, NSAIDs may not be right for you. Or if you have neuropathic pain from

damaged nerves, your doctor may turn first to adjuvant drugs like tricyclic antidepressants and seizure medications.

■ **Use pain scores as a guide.** For most treatment plans, however, the main consideration will be how intense your pain is. "If you've shattered all the bones in your face, I won't say, 'Let's start with aspirin,' " says Gitlin. Pain management often moves forward in three stages:

■ For mild pain rating 1 to 3 on a pain assessment scale, the best choice is usually an NSAID or acetaminophen.
■ For mild to moderate pain rating 4 to 6, a weak opioid such as codeine combined with an NSAID is a good pick.
■ For severe pain rating 7 or more, you may need to call on the heavy artillery of strong opioids such as morphine.

At each stage, your doctor may also prescribe an adjuvant medication like a tricyclic antidepressant, depending on your needs.

■ **Re-evaluate and reconsider.** If you're just starting a new medication or your pain has become more intense, you should check in with your doctor after 24 hours (for severe pain) to 72 hours (for mild pain). If side effects are making you miserable, your doctor can lower the dose or switch drugs. If severe pain "breaks through" your medication, your doctor may provide what's called a rescue dose of a stronger but shorter-acting drug to get you through until your regular dosage can be adjusted.

Managing Pain Without Pills

Pain drugs are usually prescribed as pills, but the oral route isn't the only way to deliver medication. In fact, there have never been more options for getting drugs—especially opioids—into your system. That's good news if you have trouble swallowing, already take too many pills, have a dry mouth, or don't easily tolerate systemic drugs that affect your entire body.

When you take narcotics orally, you might wait up to 45 minutes (depending on the formulation) for the medicine to work its way through the digestive tract and get absorbed into the bloodstream. Once it takes effect, it wears off in a matter of hours and requires a new dose. Alternative delivery systems—which some doctors count among the most important advances in pain medicine—can help you manage these pitfalls. Long-acting, sustained-release formulations of opioids—underused by doctors—are often the least invasive and most effective pain relievers. Among the options your doctor might consider:

NARCOTICS BY NEEDLE

Injection therapies—generally used in hospitals for post-op or cancer pain—are the smart bombs of pain management: Instead of carpeting the entire body with a drug in order to ease muscle, nerve, or joint pain in just one area, medicine goes precisely to the site of the pain. Injections not only tend to relieve pain faster than oral drugs (because the body doesn't have to process and absorb the drug before it will work), they deliver results at much lower doses—and thus produce fewer side effects.

Injection therapies are at the heart of patient-controlled analgesia (PCA) systems, which allow you to push a button on a small, portable device to get more painkiller when you need it through a small needle that's placed in your body. For safety, the device is programmed by your physician to limit how much medication you can take at once. Different types of injections include:

Subcutaneous. Medication is injected into the layer of fat just under the skin, often with the help of a pump that provides steady infusions of painkiller. Because they're easy to manage outside of a hospital or clinic, so-called sub-Q systems are gaining popularity.

Intravenous. Similar to subcutaneous systems and equally effective, intravenous injections place medication directly into a vein—a more precise target. Often used in hospitals, especially for cancer or post-op treatment, IVs can also be used at home, but tend to be less convenient to manage on your own than sub-Q systems.

Intraspinal. There are two kinds of injections into the spine. One, called an epidural, puts medication in the space just outside the sac that contains the spinal cord, and the other, called intrathecal administration, puts drugs inside the sac. Both methods block pain signals right where nerves are, providing significant relief with very little medication. Giving spinal injections can be delicate, however, and while pump systems are available, some doctors recommend less invasive systems for long-term treatment.

Nerve blocks. Like intraspinal injections, nerve blocks dull pain signals at or near specific nerves, either in the spine or at points in the body where pain is located. In some cases, blocking nerves can help doctors diagnose where pain originates or what kind of disorder may be causing it.

Intramuscular. For pain due to muscle spasms (often in the neck and back), injections into painfully taut areas known as trigger points can sometimes relieve pain even without a drug. In a process known as dry needling, doctors sometimes find that the irritation of the needle or an injection of saline solution makes spasms disappear, though they may return. In some cases, an anesthetic medication such as lidocaine is used for a more long-lasting effect.

Relief ▸**TIP**

A teaspoon of sugar. Not just opioid lollipops can ease your pain; the candy kind might provide some relief as well. Researchers at McGill University in Canada have found that people seem to tolerate pain better if they're sucking on something sweet—probably because the taste of sugar boosts levels of endorphins, the body's natural painkillers.

OTHER ALTERNATIVES

For all their benefits, some people find injection therapies invasive and inconvenient, which has led researchers to come up with options that fall in between pills and needles:

Skin patches. A patch system using the opioid fentanyl (Duragesic) lets medication seep slowly into the body through the skin over a period of two to three days. Though it takes 12 to 18 hours for the drug to take effect, the extended dosage provides a steady supply of painkiller without your needing to pop pills or go through a procedure to place needles. Fentanyl is hundreds of times more potent than morphine, but the slow release means you have only small amounts of the drug in your system at one time, so side effects are cut back by as much as 30 percent compared with oral opioids. One drawback: You can't control the medicine's release like you can with a PCA system, so you may need extra help managing spikes of breakthrough pain.

Lollipops. One way to deal with breakthrough pain is to suck on a lollipop containing more fentanyl, which enters the body through small blood vessels in the mucous membrane of the mouth. The lollipop briefly quells flare-ups of pain while a pill or patch continues providing steady, long-term relief.

Should You Get Surgery?

That's a tough question. Surgery can sometimes remedy conditions that cause chronic pain, such as cancer, arthritis, and disk damage in the spine. And some procedures are now being used to relieve pain by treating nerves directly. But the more extreme the solution to your pain, the more likely it is to cause complications that can offset the benefits of pain relief.

In recent years, studies have suggested that common operations for pain-causing conditions, such as joint replacement surgery to treat arthritis and spinal fusion for back pain, are no better at providing long-term pain relief than less invasive treatments like drugs. Among the reasons surgeries are risky:

- They're often irreversible
- Surgery carries a risk of infection and other side effects
- Incisions damage healthy tissue—including nerves, which can respond in unpredictable ways
- Surgery causes more acute pain—and sometimes results in long-term pain as well

Many doctors recommend having an operation for pain only as a last resort. As a rule, it is an option only if you're already on opioids, you've tried all the less invasive options, and you still find your pain unacceptable. Talk to your doctor and a specialist about operations to relieve specific conditions.

You might also ask your doctor about a procedure called neuroablation that singles out pain-causing nerves and kills them with a device that either freezes them (cryoablation) or burns them (radio frequency ablation). "These procedures are becoming more popular, but there's very little research to show which people benefit most from them and what the long-term outcomes are," says Fine of the University of Utah Pain Management Center. "Neuroablation is also very expensive, and I would approach it with caution."

Fortunately, you have other options. In fact, most pain management specialists agree that medical treatments should be used with other potent weapons against pain—from physical therapy to mental techniques that harness the power of the mind.

Back in Action

Carlos Bernardo (Herb) Treuil suspects his spirited youth might have something to do with the low-back pain that started bothering him about the time he turned 40. "I used to do barefoot and stunt water-skiing and had a couple of bad falls—and I'd had 10 car accidents before I was 21," he says.

Whatever the cause, he put up with the pain throughout his 40s, but it became worse three years ago. "It got to the point where I sometimes had to use a cane at work, and I'd spend evenings lying on the couch or on the floor just trying to find a comfortable position," says Treuil, who works in Houston. Come morning, he'd be in too much pain to stand. Instead, he would roll out of bed onto his hands and knees and crawl to a Jacuzzi in the bathroom, where he'd soak until he felt ready to get up—a process that took at least half an hour.

It all came to a head one day when Treuil was bent over a table saw. Blade whirring, a sudden spasm of pain made him jerk so violently, the saw's teeth bit into a metal slide, sending shards of metal into his forehead, lip, and chin. Finally, he went for an MRI, which revealed damaged disks and nerves in his lower spine. He slacked off walking, running, bicycling and other physical activities he enjoyed to keep his back pain from flaring. "Probably the worst thing I could have done," he says now. But nonsteroidal anti-inflammatories such as aspirin, ibuprofen, and naproxen didn't help much either—"and they tore up my stomach," he says.

At Thanksgiving two years ago, his brother-in-law, an anesthesiologist, asked how he was doing. "Rotten," Treuil told him. "He got up and wrote a prescription for a new pain drug," Treuil says. "We left the turkey on the table to get it filled at a 24-hour pharmacy." Compared to other NSAIDs, the COX-2 drug, which had just hit the market, worked a miracle: "I woke up the next day feeling 20 years younger. I felt no pain whatsoever."

With his pain under control, Treuil wasted no time signing on with a personal trainer to get himself back into physical condition, and now spends 90 minutes doing about 25 different exercises twice a week. "Once I started that, I didn't need the drug all the time," he says. He now limits his drug taking to flare-ups brought on by, for example, a recent 12-hour business flight to Buenos Aires. "Before, I couldn't stand even one hour on a plane."

The biggest benefit from quelling his pain, however, is that he can now shoot baskets with his seven-year-old son. "We just went on a camping trip," Treuil says. "I'm doing all kinds of things people with bad backs aren't supposed to be able to do."

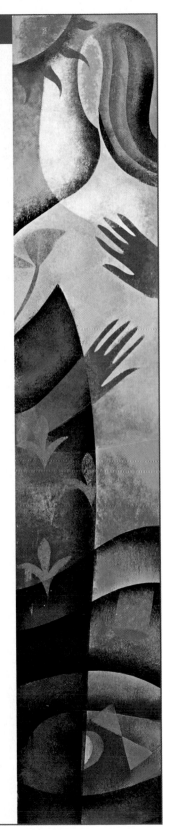

3

THE MIND-BODY ALLIANCE

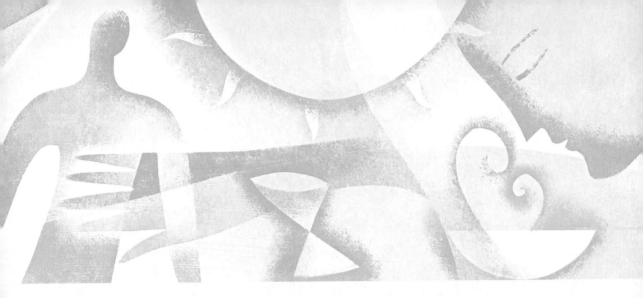

Using your mind to help you overcome pain is a satisfying way to do battle: It gives you the upper hand with minimum expense, maximum benefit, and zero negative side effects. Instead of being skeptical, your doctor will likely applaud you for your mastery of techniques that were once pooh-poohed by the medical profession. Don't leave your doctor out of the loop; good doctors today want to work with you to recapture your independence and enjoyment of life.

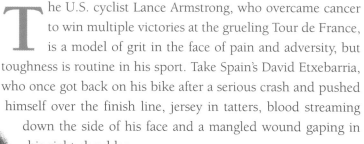

The U.S. cyclist Lance Armstrong, who overcame cancer to win multiple victories at the grueling Tour de France, is a model of grit in the face of pain and adversity, but toughness is routine in his sport. Take Spain's David Etxebarria, who once got back on his bike after a serious crash and pushed himself over the finish line, jersey in tatters, blood streaming down the side of his face and a mangled wound gaping in his right shoulder.

It almost seems as if some people don't feel pain. Think of the soldier in battle, the firefighter pulling a victim from a flaming car wreck—even the person who cheerfully endures hundreds of needle pricks and occasional cuts (without anesthesia) to get a tattoo.

The truth is that these people do feel pain—but they're concentrating on something else for a time. Researchers say these examples show that your state of mind can affect how you feel pain. "We tend to view pain as a physical experience, but you can't feel pain without the mind being involved," says Scott Fishman, M.D., chief of the division of pain medicine at the University of California, Davis, and author of *The War on Pain*. "Elite athletes find a way to tolerate negative sensations and sometimes even convert them into something positive. But you don't have to be a marathon runner to make use of mental techniques that improve your performance against pain."

What You Bring to Pain

When pain flares up, do you accept it with the unflappable serenity of a Tibetan monk? Not likely. Instead, you'll probably feel a rush of emotions: fear, anger, anxiety, and perhaps even despair. It's almost inevitable that you'll feel something—after all, pain signals from the body are channeled through the cerebral cortex and the limbic system, regions of the brain that deal with higher thinking and primal emotions.

Part of the brain's job is to decide what to make of your pain, and your emotional state can affect the brain's interpretation, actually changing the pain's intensity—or at least your perception of it. If you're stressed, tired or anxious, pain you might otherwise consider trivial can seem to hurt more. For example, a minor abdominal pain might seem barely worth your attention if you're healthy, but fear and anxiety might magnify the same pain if you think you have colon cancer. Likewise, if you're lying in the dentist's chair and dread having your cavity filled, you're more likely to jump at the slightest poke than if you feel calm, relaxed, and confident the procedure will turn out fine.

One of the most dramatic examples of the mind's power over pain was brought to light in a classic study during World War II, when a U.S. army doctor surveyed 215 soldiers who had been badly wounded during the invasion of Italy. He spoke only to those with the worst injuries, looking for ways to better treat their pain. To his surprise, when asked about their pain, 75 percent of the soldiers said they had little to none. The doctor's conclusion: Overwhelming relief at leaving the front lines and being sent home made the men euphoric, which dulled their pain.

More recently, researchers have found that even in less dramatic circumstances, a number of factors can affect your perception of pain in both good ways and bad, including:

▶ **What's happened before.** The brain draws on memory when deciding how to interpret pain, so if your pain reminds you of a previous unpleasant incident, you may feel the new pain even more strongly.

▶ **What you expect.** To some extent, pain can become a self-fulfilling prophecy. This doesn't mean you're "making up" your pain. But if you're expecting pain to be intense or debilitating, it's more likely to turn out that way. With chronic pain, anticipating months or years of ongoing discomfort can take a psychological toll that makes it difficult for more positive thoughts to keep your mind off the pain.

▶ **How much control you have.** Pain is likely to feel more oppressive if you feel you're at its command instead of the other way around. In some cases, simply having a correct

THE THREE FACES OF PAIN

As researchers unravel how pain works, they've come to recognize it has three basic components:

The sensory dimension.

This is what we normally experience as pain: the obvious, obnoxious sensations that zip through the nerves and can be described with words such as dull or sharp, deep or shallow, hot or cold.

The cognitive dimension.

This is the thinking part of pain, in which you make judgments about what your body feels, such as whether pain is harmful or harmless, irritating or aggravating, bearable or unbearable.

The motivational-emotional dimension.

This component shapes how you feel about your pain, which often depends on what's causing it. For example, you'll feel different about pain from a collision with a drunk driver (rage, resentment) than you will about pain from an accident nobody could prevent.

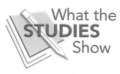

Are some groups of people more pain-tolerant than others? You'll always find variations from person to person, but studies suggest your reaction to pain is partly determined by your culture. As a result, researchers say members of certain ethnic groups seem more stoic about pain than others. For example, one recent study published in the journal *Psychosomatic Medicine* found that African Americans have more chronic pain and are more sensitive to acute pain than Caucasians. Other research shows white Anglo-Saxon women to have more tolerance to pain than (in order of highest tolerance) Jewish, Irish, and Italian women.

diagnosis or an assurance that treatment can help makes patients feel better.

▶ **How others react.** Lab studies find that people are more likely to tolerate holding on to a hot or cold object if they know other people are watching, for fear of seeming weak. Men, for example, will tolerate more if a woman is present. We take cues about how we should react to pain from watching those around us—including people we see on TV.

▶ **What else is on your mind.** When your mind is a blank slate—say, while you're lying in a dark, quiet room where nothing is happening—your brain has little to focus on besides your pain. As a result, your misery is likely to be more intense. But gabbing with a friend or filling your senses with sights and sounds makes pain compete for attention in your brain and helps push pain into the background. For example, arthritis patients report in studies that having an interesting conversation or watching an engaging movie can help ease joint pain.

At the level of nerves and brain chemicals, it's not exactly clear how thoughts and emotions might alter the pain process. The important thing is that doctors today have little doubt that mind and body are closely connected. "There's not a single class of drugs used in psychiatry that's not also used to treat pain," says Fishman. "That alone tells you there's enormous overlap between emotions and pain."

The payoff is that you can benefit from thought-based therapies that attack pain differently than drugs do. That's important in light of one recent survey that finds more than half of people taking prescription painkillers are dissatisfied with medication's effectiveness. Drugs can go a long way toward taking the edge off pain, but taking charge of your thoughts and feelings can help even more.

DRAWING THE LINE: THRESHOLD VERSUS TOLERANCE

If the mind can help control pain, does that mean you're somehow to blame if you find nagging pain tough to bear? Doctors are careful to point out that the answer is no. To understand why, it helps to know the difference between your pain threshold and your pain tolerance.

CAN PAIN BE SPIRITUAL?

It's natural to fight pain. But in many spiritual traditions around the world, people seeking higher states of being not only have embraced pain, they've made it part of their rituals.

Examples include Native Americans on the Great Plains who hung themselves by hooks in their skin, self-flagellation in medieval monasteries, and epic journeys across southern Asia by religious pilgrims who walked the entire way barefoot.

The spiritual aspects of pain are more a matter of theology than medicine. But doctors agree that, though you shouldn't seek it out, you'll find pain easier to manage if you see it as a source of insight and meaning instead of just misery. People in

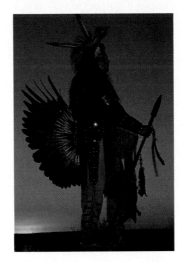

different cultures have tried to transcend suffering by believing that pain:

⚜ Increases holiness by subduing the desires of the flesh

⚜ Gives you earthly challenges that will be rewarded in the afterlife

⚜ Brings Christians closer to God by following the example of the crucified Christ

⚜ Alters your mental state, leaving you more open to mystical experiences

⚜ Provides perspective or experience that ultimately will have some positive benefit in your life, such as reuniting you with the rest of the community

Fishman suggests trying (or just thinking about) the following simple experiment to gauge your response to pain. First, fill a bowl with water and ice, then stick your hand in the frigid fluid. Count the seconds before the icy sensation becomes painful. That's your pain threshold—the point when a given stimulus starts to hurt. Next, leave your hand in the water and count the seconds until you can't take the pain anymore and have to remove your hand from the bowl. That's your pain tolerance—the point beyond your threshold when your fears, reason, and endurance make the pain unbearable for you.

Research shows that that the pain threshold tends to be about the same from one person to the next. One study, for example, found that people asked to grasp metal rods that were then heated or chilled consistently reported that the hot sensation started to hurt at 105 degrees Fahrenheit and the cold became painful at 22 degrees.

Pain tolerance, however, can vary a great deal. If you're a member of the Polar Bear Club or have a stoic personality, you may have a high tolerance for icy water. But if you were once caught outside in a blizzard and have been afraid of extreme cold ever since, your fear could magnify the pain and drive your tolerance down. In the experiment with metal rods, when participants were told that the rod's temperature would quickly cause injury, they dropped it sooner than when they weren't given this warning. In truth, the rod's temperature range always stayed the same—but anticipating harm made people less tolerant of the pain.

Mystery makes pain less tolerable. If you know your hand is going into cold water in a threshold test, you assume the water is benign. If you didn't know what the liquid was, however, you might react differently, wondering if it were dangerous. This is an issue for pain patients, who desperately seek the cause of their pain so "at least, I'll know."

THE POWER OF PLACEBOS

What if you could find a low-cost pain pill that, while not 100 percent effective, had absolutely no side effects? Would you be interested? More and more doctors are, even though the treatment in question is…no treatment at all.

Studies find that, on average, a third of patients with any given condition will get better if they're told a treatment will help—even if they're only getting a dummy pill. The figures tend to be even greater with pain sufferers, in some cases as high as 75 percent. That's why the best clinical research studies always have two groups: one that gets a real drug and one that gets a sham treatment, to control for what's known as the placebo effect.

In the past, the placebo effect was considered a nuisance—a trick of the mind or evidence of patient faking that got in the way of discovering what really works. Recently, however, doctors have been considering another view: that the placebo effect is powerful evidence of the mind's ability to ease physical suffering. In fact, placebos can sometimes produce results that rival those of real treatments.

Some doctors have gone so far as to suggest that placebos should be offered as bona fide treatments. It's a controversial idea: Many doctors feel it would be unethical to give patients empty treatments. But proponents argue no deception is needed. A doctor could simply say, "Take this pill twice a day. There's

PLACEBO PROMOTERS

Simply having a doctor take a medical history and perform an exam triggers a placebo response in some people—on top of whatever treatment the physician may recommend. Other aspects of care that can boost the mind's power over pain:

- Big pills are generally seen as more powerful than small ones
- White-colored analgesics and narcotics seem to be more powerful than colored painkillers
- Yellow seems to boost the effects of antidepressants and stimulants

no drug in it and we don't know exactly how it works, but it may stimulate the body to heal itself and your chances of improving with it are good." Some doctors speculate that alternative treatments that don't seem to have any sound medical basis may in fact be triggering a placebo response.

You may already be benefiting from mind-based pain relief Doctors find that you're probably more susceptible to placebo power when you have:

- An expectation that treatment will make you feel better
- Trust that your doctor can help you
- A willingness to try new treatments and comply with a prescription
- Anxiety about your pain—which makes you open to new sources of relief
- Severe pain, which placebos seem to affect more readily than mild pain

THE IDEAL OUTLOOK
To get a sense of how well you cope with pain, ask yourself which of these three common perspectives comes closest to how you view your suffering:

- As a punishment
- As an enemy
- As a challenge

People who view pain as a punishment tend to see themselves as victims and often fret about what they did wrong to deserve their fate.

Those who see pain as an enemy are on constant alert against a malicious foe that's always ready to strike, which can wear you down and make you feel hopeless.

Best off are those who see pain as a challenge. If you believe you can take action to control pain, you'll feel a stronger sense of control and have a more upbeat attitude. As a result, you're likely to have less depression, better coping strategies, and, ultimately, less pain.

IS PAIN "ALL IN YOUR HEAD"?
At first glance, saying that emotions help shape your pain seems to confirm what was once a common attitude: that pain may be

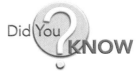

Did You **KNOW**

Placebos can work in reverse as well. Doctors report that patients sometimes suffer side effects such as gastrointestinal trouble from drugs that don't normally cause such problems—a negative turnabout sometimes called the "nocebo" effect.

all in your head—perhaps the result of hysteria, weakness, laziness, or (worst of all) a scam to get workers' compensation or narcotics. No wonder some patients bristle at the notion that the mind can help control pain. "If there's an implication that pain is a figment of the imagination, it can seem as if your doctor relinquishes responsibility to make you feel better," says Fishman, "and that's a terrifying thought." But pain experts say there's a big difference between saying that feelings count and saying that pain is fake.

"If a doctor ever doubts your pain is real, you should get out of his office and find another one," says Nelson Hendler, M.D., assistant professor of neurosurgery at Johns Hopkins University School of Medicine and clinical director of the Mensana Clinic in Stevenson, Maryland. "Some doctors still assume that pain starts with a psychological problem, especially when treatments aren't as successful as they'd like." But so-called psychosomatic pain is actually quite rare. Even when suffering has no obvious physical cause, truly "made up" pain—due to delusions or hallucinations—accounts for only an estimated 2 percent of all chronic cases.

BOTTOM LINE: Chronic pain doesn't start with emotions, it produces them. And how you handle your feelings can make a difference in how much you suffer. According to Hendler, you can expect to go through several distinct emotional stages in dealing with chronic pain as it progresses.

(1) In the first stage, which lasts about the first two months, you see your pain as acute—an irksome bother that you have every reason to expect will go away. Aside from having trouble sleeping, a well-adjusted person will generally stay that way even if pain is severe because it's easier to be upbeat and positive when you feel there's a light at the end of the tunnel.

(2) During the second stage, which goes from the second to the sixth month of pain, you start becoming more troubled. You expected the pain to end, but it didn't—what gives? Questions start to gnaw at your mind. Has something gone wrong? Did I get the right diagnosis? Did the doctor misread the X rays? Am I getting the right treatment? What can be done? At this point, you're probably still hopeful that your pain can be resolved—and you may be right. But you're probably feeling anxious and irritable, and you may start withdrawing from other people and activities that you like.

③ After six months your pain is no longer acute, it's chronic. Even if you've stayed emotionally stable so far, the thought that pain might continue well into the future can throw you into depression. Depression can make you think and talk to yourself in negative ways ("I can't work anymore, so I'm not worth anything" or "This will never change; it's hopeless") that wear you down and make pain even more difficult to fight.

④ Eventually you reach a point where you accept your pain as a reality of life. You may not be happy with your situation, but you're able to come up with strategies for coping that emphasize living with pain—and carrying on with a valuable and productive life—rather than defeating it.

At every stage, there's no denying your pain is real. In fact, the pain may not change from one stage to the next—but your emotions and your ability to cope do. Fortunately, there are steps you can take to ease your suffering when things seem at their worst.

A Toolbox of Mental Pain-Tamers

Working to change thoughts and attitudes may strike you as mind games, and maybe they are—but they're games you can play to win. Over the past several decades, researchers in the rapidly developing field known as behavioral medicine have shown that thoughts and feelings can have physical effects on the body, partly by changing how we act. Which techniques will work best for you? You can find out by trying the specific steps described below.

Mind/body pain therapies have plenty of advantages over conventional medical treatments such as drugs. (Not that they'll work miracles on their own, of course: Doctors almost always advise using them in combination with drugs and other medical treatments.) Among the advantages: Thought-based therapies usually cost little to nothing, have few (if any) nasty side effects, and can often be used without the help of a specialist—although

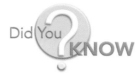

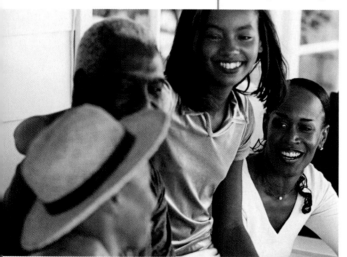

formal training is often helpful in getting you started.

Almost all mind/body pain management techniques have one purpose: to keep pain from worming itself into your thoughts. Left unchecked, constantly focusing on pain can help push you into a spiral of physical and mental debilitation. Time and again, doctors see pain take over patients' thinking about everything they do. The cycle may strike you as familiar: If you hurt, fear of more pain constrains your movement. If you don't move your body, you get out of shape. The more your physical condition declines, the more vulnerable you are to pain. Meantime, you feel bad about not doing more and begin losing your sense of self-esteem. You may stop calling on your friends, who may in turn stop calling on you. The more time you spend alone, the more you think about your pain—until soon, isolated and inactive, you find pain is all there is. Pain is in control.

But you don't have to take pain lying down. Instead, you can fight back by giving pain less of a handle on your inner life. You've taken an important first step just by reading this book: Studies find that chronically ill people do better the more they learn about their condition. "Having a clear understanding of what to expect is an important way to reduce anxiety," says Hendler. "The unknown is always most frightening." Other factors that make people better able to handle chronic illness, according to research:

- **Getting emotional support from friends and family.** Having people around to lend a hand not only helps you manage the practical tasks of daily life, it gives you a chance to talk, gain perspective from others, and feel the uplifting sense of being loved.
- **Having a supportive significant other** who distracts you without coddling and accepts your pain without ridicule or resentment.
- **Managing stress.** Stress can make pain worse in a number of ways, from promoting the sense that you're not in control to tightening muscles and making them more prone to pain.
- **Not "catastrophizing"**—as in, "This pain seems different; I

must have cancer" or "If my pain doesn't clear out by next week, I'll never work again." Always imagining the worst makes you feel even more victimized and leads to a defeated sense that nothing you do can make a difference.

■ **Not generalizing**—as in "Last time my back felt like this I needed surgery, so I must need it again now." A cousin to catastrophizing, jumping to conclusions about the future based on what's happened in the past is another way of being negative—perhaps without reason.

THE A-LIST OF CAPABLE COPING

Therapists say that most mind-based methods for mediating pain come under the umbrella of four strategies—call them the "4 A's" of successful coping.

① Avoidance

You may not be able to stop pain, but you can avoid thinking about it by exploiting a truth familiar to anyone who's ever tried multitasking: The brain can primarily focus on just one thing at a time. The more you think about something else, the less you concentrate on pain.

AVOIDANCE TECHNIQUES:
distraction, visualization, hypnosis, prayer, music therapy, laughter therapy.

② Alleviation

This method soothes pain by imagining pleasant sensations. Thinking about the comforting warmth of a hot pad on your aching back, for example, may make the brain send pain-disrupting signals to the hurting region. Some people can also use the mind to control or change how the body behaves physically.

ALLEVIATION TECHNIQUES:
progressive muscle relaxation, biofeedback, visualization, hypnosis, prayer.

③ Alteration

Some people can ease their pain by thinking about it differently. One way is to mentally convert pain to more comfortable sensations—for example, by imagining one strong pain breaking up into many smaller pains and evaporating like droplets of water. Another way is to change the meaning of the pain by imagining yourself in a different situation. For example, if you have abdominal pain, you might imagine yourself as a wartime hero who's been wounded while rescuing refugees.

ALTERATION TECHNIQUES:
hypnosis, biofeedback, visualization.

④ Awareness

A more difficult approach that takes mental discipline, awareness entails studying your pain with scientific objectivity. You might even imagine your pain as someone else's, observing from afar as if you were going to write a paper about it.

AWARENESS TECHNIQUES:
hypnosis, biofeedback, keeping a diary.

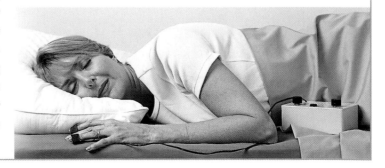

SHORT-CIRCUITING STRESS

If you're like most people, life is stressful even under the best of circumstances. Too much to do and not enough time, fear about the future, spats with family members, big changes like moving to a new home, pressure at work, dealing with responsibilities to children or parents—all can make you feel tense, tired, cranky, and anxious. But as someone with a chronic condition, you grapple with yet another major stressor: the anxiety, uncertainty, and disruption of coping with pain.

Stress is the ultimate mind/body condition: It's based on what we think and feel, but it causes obvious physical changes. When you're stressed, your body releases hormones such as adrenaline and cortisol, which trigger a remarkably wide variety of effects. Among them: Breathing becomes fast and shallow, blood pressure and heart rate shoot up, digestion slows, blood sugar rises, and you sweat more. When you're facing a real danger, these immediate effects help you confront the threat or run from it—what's known as the fight-or-flight response. Over time, however, constant stress can lead to problems like hypertension and heart disease.

Most important, stress affects pain in two critical ways: It lowers your pain threshold so your hurting seems more intense, and it tightens muscles, leaving the body more prone to pain. For example, a recent study at the University of Ohio found that stress made healthy volunteers change how they used their back muscles in a way that raised their risk of injury. Researchers also suspect that stress hinders the body's production of natural painkillers.

When you're already hurting, stress becomes a vicious circle: Pain causes stress, which makes pain worse, leading to even more stress. Add it all together and it's no wonder defusing stress is a top priority in mental management of pain.

TENSION-TAMING TACTICS

In a perfect world, you could simply avoid whatever's stressing you. But when pain and other chronic sources of tension are

---

STRESS: THE TOTAL EXPERIENCE

Stress is "holistic"—that is, it affects just about every aspect of your health and life. Here's how its symptoms affect your:

Thoughts
Stress makes you anxious about the present and fearful about the future. It also disrupts concentration, fogs memory, and hinders your ability to make decisions.

Emotions
Feeling anxious or under pressure makes you tense and unable to relax, triggers irritability, and can lead to depression.

Behavior
Stress can sap your motivation and make you prone to procrastination. It can also wreck your sleep and cause fidgeting, facial strain or grimacing, fist clenching, crying, and changes in your eating or drinking habits.

Body
In addition to tense muscles and pain (including headaches and stomachaches), stress can cause dry mouth, constipation or loose stools, and weight loss or gain.

Social life
Some people withdraw when under stress, and relationships may become strained, especially with intimate partners affected by a drop in your sex drive.

here to stay, the best approach is to take steps that focus on yourself rather than others. "Start with an attitude of patience," suggests Mark Abramson, D.D.S., who teaches two stress management courses at the Stanford University Center for Integrative Medicine and the Health Improvement Program at Stanford University Medical Center in California. "Some methods can relieve stress in minutes, but you won't be relaxed if you're feeling rushed."

Almost every mind/body therapy that reduces pain also calms stress, but you might begin by trying these steps:

○ **Snare more air.** Deep breathing almost instantly calms the body's physical response to stress, filling the lungs with oxygen, which takes strain off the heart and lowers blood pressure. Deep breathing also reduces muscle tension and helps put your mind into a state of relaxed alertness. It's easy to achieve what's known as the relaxation response by following these simple steps:

▶ Sit comfortably in a chair, keeping your torso as upright as possible.

▶ Take a deep, slow breath through your nose. (If it's more comfortable, you can also breathe through your mouth, with lips slightly parted.) Concentrate on making your belly expand—a sign you're pushing your diaphragm down, allowing your lungs to take in more air. (If only your chest expands, you're not breathing deeply enough.) "Pretend your pants are too loose and you have to expand your waistline to keep them up," Abramson suggests. Consider putting your hand on your stomach to feel whether it's expanding.

▶ Count slowly to four as you breathe in. As you count, imagine feelings of peace and serenity entering your body.

▶ Hold the breath for another slow count to four.

▶ Slowly let the air out of your lungs through either your nose or mouth while again slowly counting to four. As you exhale, imagine tension flowing out of your body with your breath.

○ **Get a move on.** You may find it tough to keep your body moving when you hurt, but it's worth making an effort to be as physically active as possible. Besides hav-

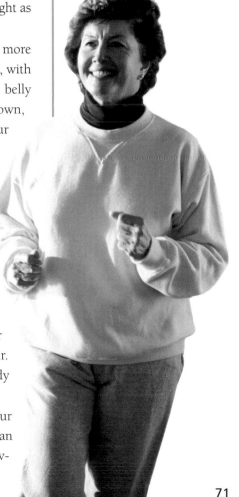

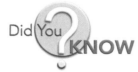

Pets such as cats and dogs can be stress busters. Research shows that being around an animal—watching it, stroking it, caring for it—can ease stress and lower blood pressure. (One caveat: If you don't like animals, all bets are off.) One study found that elderly people with pets visit the doctor less than petless peers. Another found that people released from coronary treatment at a hospital survived longer on average if they had pets.

ing physiological benefits for your body (which alone can help ease your pain; see chapter 4), exercise flushes stress hormones out of your system and relieves tension—sometimes for hours at a stretch, depending on how intensely you work out. Physical action also fosters the sense that pain doesn't rule your body, you do. By getting your body in gear, you can put some mental distance between you and your troubles, let your mind wander, and (if you're active outdoors) take in some of your natural surroundings—all of which help subdue stress.

○ **Immunize yourself.** In a form of therapy known as stress inoculation, patients use a variety of techniques to control pain and the stress it causes, including deep breathing and other relaxing strategies. But the core of the method—which you can better master with practice—is using your inner voice to calm down when pain flares up. Examples of what to tell yourself at four different stages of pain:

▶ **Preparing.** When you feel the first warning signs of approaching pain, tell yourself, "I can handle it. I've done it before. This time will be easier. Each time it happens, I learn more about coping. This will be a learning experience and I'll come away stronger."

▶ **Confronting.** When pain gets stronger, so does your determination: Say, "Pain won't get the best of me. There are plenty of things I can do to handle this—like deep breathing, turning my attention to something else, picturing a pleasant situation, or thinking of something funny."

▶ **Enduring.** When pain is at its worst, tell yourself, "Nothing lasts forever—and this won't either. I can stand it. I am strong. I'll be done with this soon enough."

▶ **Reinforcing.** When pain begins to ease off, give yourself credit for getting through it: "I stuck to my guns and stayed strong. I did well. I'll do even better next time."

○ **Seek to socialize.** When stress and pain are at their worst, you may just want to crawl under a rock. But it's usually better to look for company rather than avoid it. Studies find that surrounding yourself with caring people is one of the most effective ways to beat stress. Researchers in Europe, for example, have found that people speaking off the cuff or doing mental math in front of an audience have fewer stress hormones in their blood if a friend is in the audience. Social support makes you feel less isolated, boosts self-esteem, takes your mind off pain, and makes you feel more in control of your life.

DRIVEN TO DISTRACTION

One of the most basic mental management methods is to take your mind off your pain—literally, by focusing your thoughts on ideas, activities, or sensations that will compete with pain for attention in the brain. Known as distraction, the technique can be used in a variety of ways, depending on how your mind works. For example, people have been known to ease pain by doing calculus proofs in their heads. Not your idea of a pleasant diversion? Try reading, watching television, going to the theater, playing computer games, chatting on the Internet, doing crossword puzzles, playing chess, working on a hobby or craft anything you enjoy counts. If you're still at a loss for what to do, try these suggestions:

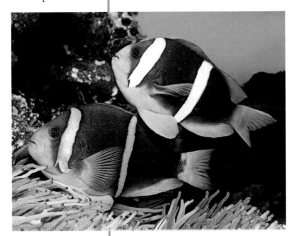

- ▷ **Go fish.** Research shows that people who stare into the placid waters of an aquarium stocked with vibrant tropical fish, plants, and rocks quickly become transfixed by the movement, color, and gentle bubbling. The effect is strong enough to make people enter a calm and relaxed state that can actually make blood pressure drop from elevated levels to the normal range—effects that aren't seen when subjects gaze into an empty tank of water.

- ▷ **Find your comfort zone.** If one part of your body is hurting, don't focus your attention there. Instead, scan your body for places that *aren't* in pain. Concentrate on all the sensations you feel in one pain-free area—say, your mouth, which is exceptionally sensitive. Take notice of how your tongue, saliva, teeth, gums, and oral cavity feel. Move your tongue around, focusing all your awareness on the quality of its touch. Put a chocolate or succulent fruit in your mouth and savor its sensation and flavor.

- ▷ **Follow your nose.** The sense of smell is thought to soothe the brain's limbic system, which is also involved with processing pain signals. Although more research needs to be done on how smells may ease pain, simply focusing on olfactory sensations can conjure up memories and emotions that carry your mind away. One study in which people were exposed to different odors while responding to stress-producing questions found that the scent of spiced apple relaxed muscles, lowered blood pressure, and slowed breathing.

▶ **Take charge with touch.** Use your hands to direct your thoughts using a form of distraction (sometimes used in hypnosis) known as the tactile-kinesthetic method. It's easier than it sounds. First, focus your attention on one of your hands. Gently rub your fingers together, concentrating on all the sensations you feel. Pay attention to tactile qualities such as texture and temperature. Try the same exercise on the other hand and try to identify differences (a scab, dryness, a wart) between the two hands. Another touch distraction is to make a fist with the fingers of one hand. Clench your fist as tightly as possible, then squeeze tighter. Feel the tension it produces in your hand and arm. Now release your fist and feel the tension flowing out. Picture your pain being released with the tension.

▶ **Look around.** Gaze at your surroundings. Pick a single area or object and imagine you're going to paint or draw it. Take note of all its subtleties—the wood grain and color of a table, the pattern of a sofa, the cut of a tile floor.

▶ **Stroll your home.** If sitting and looking seems too passive, take your shoes off and move from room to room. Pay attention to each footfall and how the textures of different floorings—carpet, vinyl, tile, wood—feel on the soles of your feet.

TAKING A MENTAL VACATION

A second way to take your mind off pain is similar to distraction, but doesn't rely on outward sights and sensations. Instead, it taps the power of your imagination to take your mind someplace else. Known as imagery, or visualization, this method might seem a pale substitute for the actual happenings that make distraction work. But imagery may be even more potent than distraction because it requires greater mental effort, better loosening pain's grip on your thoughts. Athletes use it to train, visualizing every detail of a successful race or ski run. The most basic form of imagery is daydreaming, which can help keep pain in the shadows. But willfully directing your thoughts in a more disciplined way can make pain less likely to intrude uninvited on your mind. There's nothing difficult about imagery: You can take yourself to whatever place or time you find most pleasant or interesting. One key to bear in mind: Don't just think in pictures. Instead, think sensuously. The more you conjure up sensory details—sounds, smells, tastes, as well as sights—the better you'll be able to distance yourself from pain.

Ask your doctor for guided visualization exercises on audiotape or look for such tapes at a bookstore. To get started, try these mental exercises on your own.

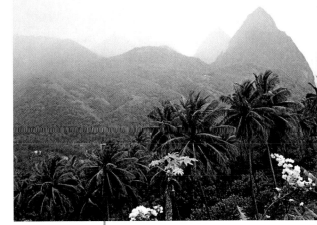

■ Exercise A

Take an imaginary journey to a place brimming with natural beauty and a variety of sensations. Imagine yourself at the top of a mountain high above a tropical rain forest. There's a clear blue sky, the sun is shining, and you can feel its warmth on your skin. The air is fresh with the fragrance of brightly colored flowers and the smell of newly fallen rain, which glistens on the foliage. You can hear birds singing and insects buzzing. A gentle breeze blows, and far below, you can see palm trees of the forest meeting an expanse of an empty white beach on a lake.

■ Exercise B

Move to another beautiful setting, perhaps as an extension of the previous exercise. Picture yourself walking along the beach of a lake, the soft sand under your bare feet making a whispering sound with your steps. The air is gentle and warm, and waves lap gently at the shore. You're completely alone and at peace. You see a boat moored at the shore, the waves slapping quietly at its stern. You get into the boat and find soft, warm blankets inside. Untying the boat, you lie on the blankets and gently drift under puffy white clouds. A deep sense of relaxation comes over you as the water gently rocks you. You hear the sound of the water, see the clouds scuttling across the blue, feel the warmth of the sun, smell the moist air scented with flowers from the shore.

■ Exercise C

On this exercise, try filling in some of the details on your own. Picture yourself sitting at a table. Imagine what the table looks like—what it's made of, its color, its texture. Picture the chair. Does it match the table? Is it hard or soft? Does it make you sit high or low?

On the table you see a white plate. It's so clean, it sparkles. Imagine touching the plate and feeling its silky smooth texture.

Next to the plate is a knife. Imagine its size. What does the handle look like? How is it shaped? What color is it? You gingerly touch the blade with your finger. Is it serrated or smooth? How sharp does it seem?

On the plate is a large whole lemon. Picture touching the lemon, feeling its smoothly pitted skin. How does it nestle in your hand? How heavy does it feel? Can you smell it?

You pick up the knife. Grasping the lemon, you cut through its skin with the knife. Imagine the sensation of the juice seeping onto your fingers—its temperature, its stickiness. Picture smelling the citrus aroma. Mentally raise the lemon to your nose and take a deep whiff.

Cut a slice of the lemon and touch your tongue to it. Do you like the taste of raw lemon? Is the sour sensation mild or overpowering? Take a bite of the lemon, letting the juices flow into your mouth. Imagine the texture of the fruit in your mouth. Picture swallowing the bite. How does your mouth feel? Look back at the lemon—and decide if you want more.

THE RELIEF OF RELAXATION

Studies suggest that mental relaxation therapies may directly reduce pain—perhaps because pain-causing conditions such as irritable bowel syndrome, headaches, and muscle spasms are often triggered by tension. But even when pain isn't directly tied to those kinds of problems, relaxation therapies seem to quell pain. It stands to reason: If you're relaxed, you're less stressed. In one University of Mississippi study, for example, 60 percent of headache patients cut their pain by at least half when they

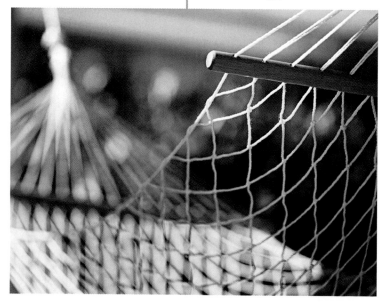

practiced relaxation techniques along with cognitive behavioral therapy (in which they identified and controlled negative feelings). Studies at Duke University find that relaxation therapy can ease low back pain.

The first step in most relaxation techniques is to do deep breathing (p.73). From there, you can move to the following methods:

● **Body scan.** With this technique, let your mind rove over every part of your body to search out areas of tension and mentally focus on relaxing them. Here's how it works:

▶ As you breathe in, concentrate on a specific part of your body, starting with the forehead. Take note of how much tension you feel in that area.

▶ As you breathe out, consciously relax the targeted muscles, letting tension flow out of them. Keep doing this for several deep breaths.

▶ Concentrate on another area of your body, moving next to the muscles around the eyes. After that, focus on the mouth and jaw, neck, back (all the way down the spine), shoulders, upper arms, lower arms, hands, chest, and stomach.

▶ When you've finished the upper body, do another quick forehead-to-waist scan to identify any lingering tension.

▶ Move on to the lower body, starting with the pelvis and buttocks, then proceeding to the upper legs, lower legs, ankles, and feet.

▶ To conclude, do a mental check of your entire body to find and release all areas of tension.

● **Progressive muscle relaxation.** Sometimes abbreviated PMR, progressive muscle relaxation goes a step beyond the body scan. Instead of simply releasing the tension in a certain area, you begin by first making the area more tense. The reason: Most people can't tell whether muscles are tense just by thinking about them. Accentuating the tension makes it easier to gauge how tight an area is so the process of release seems even more relaxing. To do it:

▶ Again, start with the forehead. Make your muscles as tight as you can for a slow count of five.

Relief ▶**TIP**

For a quick and easy way to tune out tension, here's a technique you can count on: Consider your body's tension a 10 on a scale running from 0 to 10. Now count backward from 10, letting your body become more relaxed as you mentally hit each number. Breathe deeply and take it slowly, saying each number as you exhale, releasing more tension with every breath.

▶ Let go of the tension while deeply breathing in.

▶ Repeat the process in the same region, then move on to the next. For each area, tense muscles twice before letting all tightness flow out of them.

When you come to areas that are in pain, don't tense muscles if it will make you hurt more. Instead, skip the PMR and use the basic body scan technique.

▶ **The autogenic appeal.** To use a form of relaxation therapy called autogenic training, try progressively concentrating on different parts of the body as you do with a body scan. But instead of consciously releasing tension, repetitively make statements suggesting heaviness and warmth in the selected area. For example, while focusing on the shoulders, you might simply say, "My shoulders are heavy and warm. My shoulders are getting heavier and warmer." Fans of the method, developed by a German psychiatrist and hypnotist, say such straightforward statements boost blood flow to targeted areas, reduce pain, and promote well-being.

MAKING THE MOST OF MEDITATION

Meditation has been part of spiritual practices all over the world for thousands of years, but even if you're not exactly seeking enlightenment, you can use its basic techniques to calm your body, ease your mind, and tame your pain. Meditation isn't difficult in theory. In fact, the whole point is to keep your thinking simple by focusing all your attention on one or two things: your breathing and, typically, a meaningful word or phrase—what's known as a mantra. The hard part is keeping all the other thoughts that zing through your head from intruding on your single-minded focus. If you have trouble at first, don't sweat it. Just recognize distracting (and probably stressful) thoughts for what they are, let them pass through your mind, and refocus on your mantra. Here's how to have a successful session:

1. Set aside at least 10 minutes in a quiet, comfortable place where you will not be disturbed.

2. Choose a simple, calming word or phrase to focus on. Many people use words they find religiously significant, such as "shalom," "the Lord

is my shepherd," or "hail Mary," but you can also use neutral words like "peace."

③ Start by taking about 10 deep breaths. Keep your eyes closed, or focus on a single object such as a lighted candle or a stone.

④ As you continue breathing deeply, silently repeat your mantra. Try not to judge whether your meditation is "working" or not. Just keep focused on your breathing and your mantra, letting yourself become increasingly relaxed.

POLLYANNA POWER

The tale of Pollyanna gets a bad rap as a shallow, syrupy fable that tells us putting on a happy face will make the world perfect. But in the real story, a positive outlook doesn't spare Pollyanna from pain and suffering, it helps her and others cope. The essence of her optimism is a technique that cognitive behavior psychologists call "reframing." The idea isn't to delude yourself with false, chirpy platitudes, but to challenge negative, irrational thoughts that can drag you down and replace them with more upbeat thoughts that in many cases are actually more realistic:

> ### SELF-HELP RESOURCES
>
> Most bookstores have an audiotape section that features self-help titles for hypnosis, guided imagery, visualization, and relaxation techniques. Video stores (and libraries) stock a variety of therapeutic exercise tapes and CDs.

① The first step is to recognize what you tell yourself when pain or stress flares up. For example, you may find yourself thinking, "I'm miserable and it's never going to change."

② Next, ask yourself pointed questions. Is what you're thinking true? Is it logical? Does it make you feel more stressed?

③ Now try to frame your feelings differently. Think in terms of action, and try to be assertive. For example, you might say, "I'm not feeling great today, but there's plenty I can do to feel better tomorrow," or "These negative thoughts are just making things worse. I need to find something to distract me."

THE BENEFITS OF BIOFEEDBACK

Without biofeedback, mind/body medicine might never have gotten off the ground. It started in the 1970s, when almost nobody (at least in the medical establishment) questioned the long-held belief that the physical and psychological realms were distinct and separate. Then came studies showing that rats could be trained to change their heart rates and blood pressure to get food. Scientists soon discovered they could get people to do the same thing—not for food, but to relieve headaches and symptoms of other conditions.

Biofeedback is like relaxation therapy with a technical twist: Special equipment lets you know whether your body is doing what your mind wants. To use biofeedback, you typically go into a quiet room where electrical sensors are taped to various parts of your body. The sensors send information to a monitor that gives you "feedback" such as beeps or graphs indicating your skin temperature, muscle tension, heartbeat, breathing, brain waves, or sweat production, depending on the setup.

Biofeedback is often used to treat muscle spasms, headaches, stress, anxiety, and cardiovascular conditions. At first, it takes training and practice (not to mention equipment). Ask your doctor to recommend a practitioner who can get you started. After you gain experience, you'll be even more skilled at mentally controlling your body on your own.

HARNESSING HYPNOSIS

Chances are, your image of hypnosis is of people becoming entranced by a swinging pocket watch or induced to cluck like chickens in front of a live audience. Indeed, hypnotism has been fodder for dramas, parlor tricks, and comedy routines almost from the time it was developed in the eighteenth century by the Austrian physician Franz Anton Mesmer. (His name is the basis for the term "mesmerize.") But Mesmer was interested in using hypnotism to treat medical problems—and today, his methods are gaining surprising credibility as treatments for a range of conditions including hypertension, anxiety, insomnia, and obesity.

Most important, some people find hypnosis to be a potent pain reliever. One review of 27 different experiments involving a total of 933 subjects found that hypnosis relieved pain in an impressive 75 percent of cases. In some people, hypnotism's pain-easing power matched or beat that of morphine. Other studies have shown that women with advanced breast cancer need less pain medication and survive longer when they practice self-hypnosis. It's more than just a placebo effect: Research finds that the pain-relieving effects of hypnosis are three times

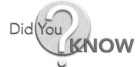

Did You **KNOW**

Hypnotism can be so effective at relieving pain, it's been used by dentists and other doctors as the sole anesthesia in procedures on people who can't tolerate chemical painkillers.

stronger than that of a sugar pill.

Scientists are baffled about how hypnosis works, but speculate that being guided to pain relief while in a trance somehow uses higher brain functions to override pain signals. Not everyone can be hypnotized: Some people are more "suggestible" than others. But people whose minds seem open to hypnosis find it remarkably easy to fall into a hypnotic trance in which they're aware of their surroundings but can respond to suggestions from a therapist. (Contrary to popular belief, hypnosis can't make you do things you'd normally avoid or give you abilities you don't already possess.) Best of all, hypnosis appears to be harmless.

While you can learn to put yourself into a state of hypnosis, you will need a trained therapist to evaluate your susceptibility (typically using a benchmark called the Stanford Hypnotic Susceptibility Scales) and get you started. To find a therapist, contact the National Board for Certified Clinical Hypnotherapists, Inc., at 800-449-8144 or online at www.natboard.com.

THE SOUND OF RELIEF

Music combines elements of a number of mind/body pain-relief techniques: It distracts your attention, creates mental images, boosts your mood, reduces stress, and can compel you to move your body. Who knows—if the beat's hypnotic, it may even throw you into a trance. (Some hypnotherapists find that just the simple beat of a metronome can induce hypnosis.)

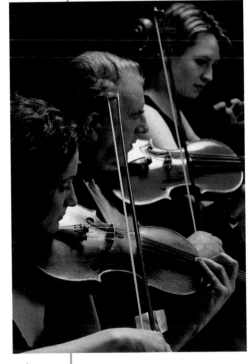

Researchers have found that music can bring down blood pressure, slow the heart, ease pain, and even reduce the amount of anesthesia needed for surgery or dental work. (It's no accident that your dentist plays soothing melodies as you lie in the chair.) The effect is particularly strong when you're able to choose the tunes yourself.

Some pain treatment centers employ music therapists, who typically choose music based on your temperament and mood. For example, if you're melancholy, you might be given music in a minor key, along with selections that can steer your mood in a more upbeat direction. But you certainly don't need special help choosing music that touches you or engages your imagination. The most appealing style of music will vary from one person to the next, but most people find slow, quiet instrumental music most calming. Just be sure to give the soothing strains your full concentration: Music won't have any therapeutic value if it's just background noise while you concentrate on something else.

LAUGHTER AS MEDICINE

It's tough to feel pain and suffering when you're laughing—just as it's tough to laugh when you're in pain. But tickling your funny bone even when you're suffering may benefit your health and ease pain. In one recent study, researchers at Loma Linda University in California found that people who watched a video of a comedy routine (the funnyman Gallagher smashing fresh produce with a sledgehammer) showed significant

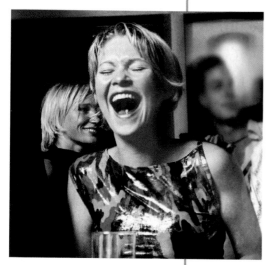

improvement in immune system functions such as natural killer cell activity. Other studies have had similar results. In one, just anticipating a humorous video boosted subjects' moods and made them less tense.

Meanwhile, around the globe, chapters of an organization called the World Laughter Tour are springing up to promote "therapeutic laughter" exercises that don't involve joke-telling or funny stories. In one typical workout, participants clap their hands in a 1-2, 1-2-3 pattern while saying the words, "Ho-ho, ha-ha-ha." Other activities involve stretching and actions borrowed from yoga.

Participants say such exercises promote deep breathing, raise spirits, and promote a sense of well-being— all of which could help ease pain. (To find a Laughter Tour chapter near you, call 800-669-5233 or log on to www.world-laughtertour.com.)

It's possible the act of laughing has benefits apart from humor. It is known, for example, as a stress reliever, and people who laugh readily are less likely to have coronary heart disease than those who are less apt to chuckle at life's endless ironies. But researchers who study laughter for itself say the real payoff for most people comes from enjoying the company of others—making laughing with friends a form of social support with extra benefits.

Thinking Through Pain

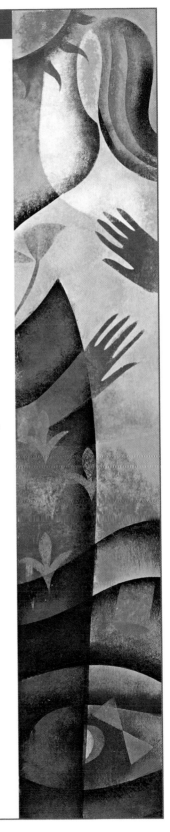

Doctors still can't explain what happened to Diane Kriemelmeyer in 1991. She says something hit her with "a sudden, massive, neurological impact." One theory is that her central nervous system was stricken with a virus. "I've been worked up for everything from multiple sclerosis to Parkinson's disease," she says, "but nothing explained what happened to me."

She lost strength and function in both her legs, suffered from tremors, and had spasms, especially in her legs, in which muscles contracted—"and wouldn't let go," she says. "It was extremely painful." Similar spasms in her back on top of degenerative disk disease in her spine also caused severe low-back pain. She was confined to a wheelchair for 10 years while she sought relief. By 2001, Kriemelmeyer was on a dozen different medications antidepressants, anticonvulsants, and opioid painkillers.

Then one of her doctors referred her to a chronic pain treatment program in the department of psychiatry and behavioral medicine at Johns Hopkins University School of Medicine in Baltimore. She spent four weeks in an inpatient program that put her on a demanding schedule of treatment by a doctor, occupational and physical therapists— and a variety of classes, group sessions, and mind/body therapies. The physical results are impressive: By the time Kriemelmeyer was discharged, she had moved from her wheelchair to a walker, crutches, a cane, and finally to her own two feet.

But, she says, "the biggest change was learning how to control my response to pain rather than just reacting to it so it controlled me." She was particularly struck by biofeedback. "When hooked to the electrodes, I could watch a line on a computer screen actually show how my mind was making my muscles relax. It was very compelling."

Now she's able to use other techniques that have proved just as effective, including progressive muscle relaxation and visualization. Cognitive therapy taught her to control unhelpful thinking. "If you're having a bout of insomnia, negative thoughts like 'I'll never get to sleep!' just automatically pop up," she says. "We used a worksheet to identify thoughts like that and correct them—'I'm going to sleep eventually; everyone does.' "

Kriemelmeyer now controls her pain without medication. On a scale of 10, her pain has gone from an average of a 6 to a 2. "I've gone from being a stay-at-home to being very involved with the world again," she says. "I'm on the board at my condominium, I'm going to night school to add a teaching certificate to my bachelor's degree, and I'm leading a much more normal life."

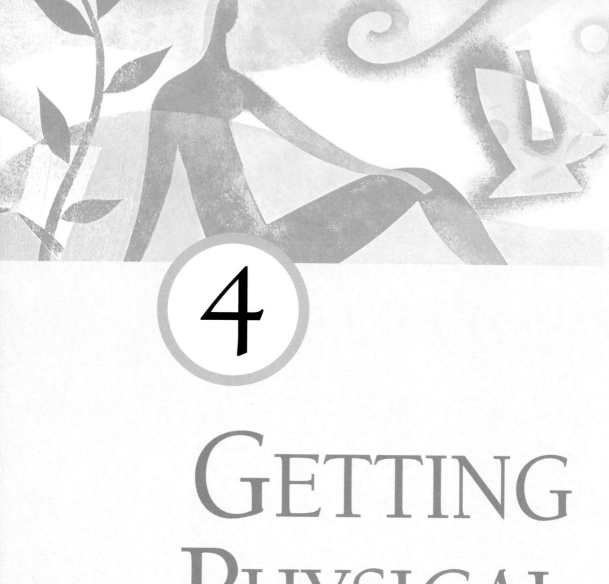

4

GETTING
PHYSICAL

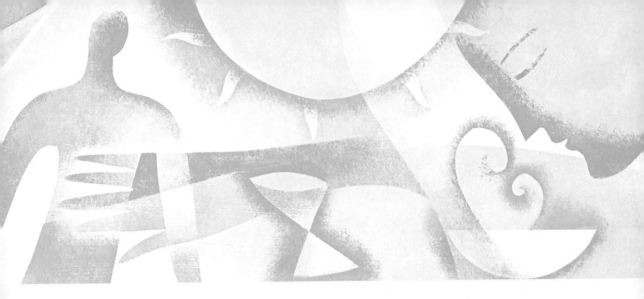

It's not magic, but physical therapy—exercises, massage, whirlpools, electrical stimulation, and ultrasound, to name a few possibilities—can not only decrease your pain, but also make you stronger and more lithe, whatever your chronic problem or your age. Building back up a pain-wracked body helps protect you from future bouts of agony, too. Let a physical therapist show you how to do the correct exercises at home; then learn a moving meditation discipline like yoga or t'ai chi from a good teacher for peace of mind and body.

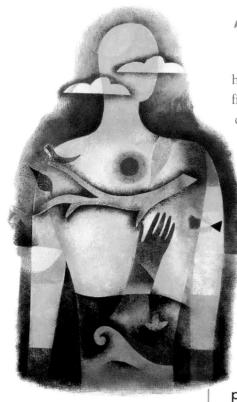

Taking pain-relieving medications? Check. Using your mind to help subdue your suffering? Check. Still have pain? For many, that's a distinct possibility. But take heart: You haven't exhausted all your options. In addition to fine-tuning what you're already doing, there's a third major component of many pain-relief programs that you can turn to: the body itself.

It's the flip side of the mind/body equation. Yes, your thoughts, attitudes, and emotional state can affect how you physically perceive pain. But the ways you move, manipulate, and carry your body can also be critically important for easing discomfort, healing injuries, and lifting the burden of pain from your mind.

Fighting Back with Physical Therapy

The main weapon in the body-based battle against pain is physical therapy, or PT. Broadly speaking, physical therapy refers to any non-drug program that works to restore the body to its pre-pain condition. PT uses an impressive variety of techniques that can not only help quell your pain, but rejuvenate your body so that it's less liable to hurt. At its most successful, PT can actually make the body stronger and more resilient than it's been in years.

"Relieving pain is the first goal of physical therapy, but it's only a start," says Richard Materson, M.D., clinical professor of physical medicine and rehabilitation at the University of Texas Medical School and Baylor College of Medicine, and vice president of medical development for Memorial Hermann Healthcare System in Houston. "Once pain is under control, you can start working to enhance your overall function."

Overall function is an issue, because when you're in pain, your body suffers in ways that can go far beyond the pain itself. Even a pain that lasts for just a short time makes you carry your body differently. It's natural: You want to avoid movements or positions that make pain worse, so you limp, slouch, guard your muscles—whatever it takes to keep the sizzle or ache at bay. The problem is, this can cause a domino effect of physical reactions throughout your body. For example, if you limp to keep pressure off a bum knee, you'll put new pressure on the other knee, which may soon start hurting as well, which changes your gait, which puts extra strain on your hips … and so it goes.

Physical therapy tries to break the cycle of pain-upon-pain by focusing on a number of goals:

- **Reducing pain.** Ultimately, of course, physical therapy is meant to relieve pain over the long haul. But it's important to first tackle pain you're feeling here and now so you're physically comfortable participating in the body-bolstering therapy to come. If you're already using medication and mind/body methods, PT has its own techniques for easing pain.

- **Restoring normal motion.** If your posture or movements are out of whack because of pain, getting back to more natural patterns is a top priority. In many cases, a slow buildup of tension from improper body mechanics is what triggered pain in the first place. Physical therapy helps you get muscles, tendons, and ligaments moving through their full range of motion, which prevents them from causing unnatural strain or tension, and makes you less vulnerable to pain and injury.

- **Building strength.** When you're dealing with chronic pain, you may not feel much like getting exercise. But keeping muscles active keeps them strong. Strong muscles gird and support pain-prone areas of the body, such as the back and joints, and make it easier for you to take on normal tasks—working in the garden, climbing a flight of stairs, or tying your shoes.

- **Boosting endurance.** As you restore normal movement and firm up your muscles, you can start getting your entire body in better condition. It's common to get out of shape when sidelined with chronic pain. But simple exercises like walking can strengthen your cardiovascular system and tone muscles, further bolstering your resistance to pain.

- **Increasing self-confidence.** Physical therapy is a form of behavioral therapy. Patients see by their own accomplishments—more strength, higher endurance, greater range of motion—that they can succeed at difficult tasks.

Physical therapy may not be appropriate for every type of pain. Some doctors, for example, feel PT does little to relieve pain from compressed or damaged nerves. But even in these cases, physical therapy isn't likely to be harmful, and may prevent musculoskeletal pain from flaring up due to poor posture.

A Note of Caution. Much of physical therapy is blessedly low-tech, using only the natural forces of your own body or another person's healing touch. But properly using exercise, stretching, and other techniques to heal pain isn't always as simple as it looks. PT should be supervised healing. That means you, working with your doctor, should seek expert advice, guidance, and hands-on treatment from a professional physical therapist. A physical therapist can evaluate your condition and put together a program that will best meet your needs. With some treatments, you might also benefit from a specialist trained in a particular technique such as massage, yoga, or various forms of bodywork. Once you get going—with your doctor's okay—you'll probably be able to use a variety of therapies on your own.

Running Hot and Cold

The age-old standbys of heat and cold are still among the first and foremost pain-taming tools that physical therapists recommend. Temperature change works on your body the same way it works on anything else: Cold tends to make things constrict, while heat tends to make things expand. That generally makes cold good for shrinking swelling and reducing inflammation, while heat is ideal for boosting blood flow and making muscles relax.

Beyond these physical effects, cold and heat help close the gate on pain signals by making nerves focus on a sensation other than pain. You can use cold and heat to relieve pain either separately or together. In fact, alternating between hot and cold is often more soothing than either method would be alone. Which approach you use depends on your condition. Here's what you need to know.

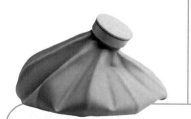

MIXING HOT AND COLD

Alternating hot and cold produces a "milking" effect that helps move metabolic wastes such as lactic acid out of aching muscles, reduces swelling, and eases pain in joints. One way to switch-hit:

▷ Apply a hot pad or moist, heated towel to a pain site such as an aching joint for three to four minutes.

▷ Remove the heat and give treatment a rest for one minute.

▷ Apply an ice pack to the same site for one minute.

▷ Repeat several times, ending with heat.

GIVING PAIN THE COLD SHOULDER

Cold is most often used for acute pain following an injury such as a cut, sprain, or blow that could lead to bruising. But many people find cold (sometimes called cryotherapy) useful for chronic pain as well. One reason: In addition to shrinking blood vessels and tissues at an injury site and distracting you from pain, cold actually makes nerves conduct pain signals more slowly to the brain.

The numbing of cold is especially good for the inflammatory pain of rheumatoid arthritis, but it's also often used for pain following surgery, headaches, minor burns, dental pain, and a variety of other conditions. You can also use cold after exercising to soothe overworked muscles or speed recovery from overuse injuries such as shinsplints or tennis elbow.

Although you can buy freezer-ready gel packs that easily mold to the contours of your skin, treating yourself with ice doesn't demand any special equipment. To make an ice pack, fill a plastic zip-lock bag with ice from your freezer and place it on the area that hurts. (You can also use a pack of frozen peas or berries.) Just be sure to wrap the ice pack in a towel to keep frostbite from damaging your skin. Check your skin regularly and avoid holding ice on any one area for more than 15 or 20 minutes at a time.

TURNING UP THE HEAT

Anyone who's soaked in a steamy bath knows heat can be deeply relaxing, and that alone can take the edge off pain. But heat also dilates blood vessels, which boosts circulation. More blood flow brings extra oxygen and nutrients to areas that need repair, along with healing substances such as waste-scavenging white blood cells and natural anti-inflammatory pain relievers such as cortisone. Another plus: "If you're taking an NSAID medication, heat will help it reach your pain more quickly," says Materson. Heat is often used for general aches, especially in the neck and lower back, but it also helps relieve deeper pain in joints and muscles.

You can take your heat either dry (from lamps, electric heat-

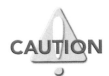

CAUTION

Because constricting arteries and veins can slow blood flow and potentially raise blood pressure, you should avoid using cold therapy if you have conditions marked by poor circulation, such as peripheral vascular disease or diabetes mellitus.

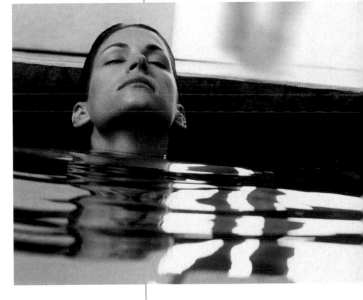

ing pads, or sunlight) or moist (from hot baths, showers, or water bottles), but most people find that moist heat penetrates best. Even so, all these methods are considered superficial—that is, close to the body's surface—and have trouble reaching pain that's more than skin-deep. Fortunately, it's possible to turn up the thermostat on pain in deeper muscles, joints, tendons, and bones through a treatment (available from your doctor or a specialist) known as diathermy, which delivers heat using ultrasound, microwave, or shortwave radiation.

Another way to ease pain with heat is to rub on topical creams such as Ben-Gay or Aspercreme. Though many of these ointments contain salicylates, a class of anti-inflammatory pain relievers that includes aspirin, some experts feel their effectiveness comes from the warmth you feel on your skin.

HYDRO-HEALING

Water has been used to heal illnesses and ease pain for thousands of years. The ancient Greek physician Galen made baths an integral part of his treatments, and cold baths became the height of fashion in ancient Rome after Emperor Augustus claimed they cured a mysterious disease that resisted other

Relief ▶TIP

Moist heat trick. To whip up a pad of penetrating moist heat, sprinkle a towel with water until it's slightly damp, fold it over, and place it in a microwave oven. Set the timer on high for one minute. Then, making sure it's not too hot to handle, place the towel on your aching muscles.

WAYS WATER CAN HELP

	Relieves joint and muscle pain	Eases tension and anxiety	Soothes foot pain	Relieves hemorrhoids and anal fissures	Increases strength and mobility
Hot shower	X	X			
Hot or cold compresses	X				
Warm bath	X	X	X	X	
Alternating hot and cold soak or shower	X		X		
Whirlpool	X	X	X		
Water exercises	X	X			X
Steam	X	X			
Sitz bath				X	

remedies. Today, spas and natural hot springs continue attracting people for their curative powers. Some enthusiasts call water our oldest natural medicine.

Not surprisingly, water is a basic part of physical therapy as well. Technically known as hydrotherapy, water treatments take a variety of forms, such as bubbling whirlpools, pulsating showers, steamy saunas, hot or cold compresses, and sitz baths. Exercising in water can help restore muscle tone and range of motion while putting a minimal amount of stress on joints, bones, and other parts of the body.

Some therapists say that water refreshes the spirit as well as rejuvenates the body. There's no doubt water has special appeal to most people, but many of water's healing effects are probably due to its value as a medium for heat and cold, massage, and pain-blocking stimulation of nerve endings in the skin.

The Suppleness Solution

Chances are, you could stand to become more limber even if you weren't in pain: Age-related declines in flexibility start kicking in as early as the teens—well ahead of other physical declines. When you're in pain, being able to move muscles and joints through their full range of motion is even more important: It's the key to getting your body mechanics back on track and building toward a future with less discomfort.

Even though flexibility is an essential part of basic fitness, it's often overlooked. Ironically, that's good news: While flexibility usually declines by about 5 percent per decade, most resilience loss is due to simple neglect, which means a program of regular stretching can undo years of built-up stiffness. If you're not familiar with the fundamentals of flex, that's okay: A physical therapist can guide you in choosing appropriate stretches and exercises, but there's a lot you can do to expand your body's mobility on your own.

Keeping yourself limber not only protects against pain from tight muscles, it keeps that tightness from spreading to other areas of the body. For example, tight calves can trigger pain in

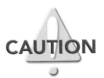

CAUTION

To sidestep potential health hazards and keep yourself from getting burned when using heat, don't combine heat treatment such as a hot-water bottle with an over-the-counter ointment that also heats the skin: The combination may cause a burn. Also, set electric hot pads on low or medium rather than high. And check with your doctor before using heat if you have pain from:

> an acute injury that makes you bleed or bruise (heat can make bleeding worse)

> cancer (heat may speed the growth of a malignancy)

> a condition such as diabetes (which can make you lose sensation, hindering your ability to detect a burn)

the knees, shins, and feet. Beyond that, restoring flexibility throughout your body keeps imbalances in check. For instance, if you have a tight hamstring in one leg, but not the other, that can make your thigh muscles work harder to keep the body properly aligned, which can trigger pain in your knees.

HOW TO STRETCH YOURSELF

Improving pliability isn't difficult—in fact, stretching is probably the easiest part of any exercise program. Still, it's important to understand a few basic concepts. First, you're working against a natural tendency for muscles to contract, so stretching has to be done regularly to have much effect. Contracting, or shortening, is how muscles exert force and perform work, whether it's lifting an item to a shelf or strolling down the sidewalk. Stretching has the opposite goal: lengthening muscles. By consistently pulling muscles slightly beyond their normal length, you gradually enable them to expand their range of motion.

You and your physical therapist can choose from a number of different stretching techniques, but the simplest and safest form is known as static stretching. Static stretches are done slow and easy, using small amounts of force usually provided by a combination of gravity and your own body weight. To make stretches both safe and effective, you need to follow some fundamental rules.

PLIABILITY PLUSES

If you're trying to regain your flexibility as part of a regular on-going exercise program, stretching may also benefit you by:

▣ Reducing soreness after you finish a workout

▣ Helping muscles feel less tired by clearing them of metabolic waste products such as lactic acid

▣ Improving muscle balance and coordination

▣ Making muscles stronger by allowing them to exert force through a greater range of motion

- **Give muscles a head start.** When muscles are cold, they're stiffer. Starting out with 5 to 10 minutes of easy activity such as slow walking (just enough so you're on the verge of breaking a light sweat) warms muscles up and makes them more pliable even before you begin stretching.
- **Move gently.** Stretching is not a speedy form of exercise. Keep the pace slow and relaxed, and keep your movements under control at all times to avoid tearing or straining muscles by stretching them too far.
- **Feel the tug.** With each exercise, ease into the stretch until you feel a gentle tug of resistance, which marks the extent of the muscles' normal range of motion. Stretch slightly beyond that point so it begins to feel mildly uncomfortable—but no further.
- **Hold for 30 seconds.** Stretched muscles aren't inactive: When lengthened beyond their normal range, they automatically react to prevent injury by shortening—an involuntary response known as the stretch reflex. To overcome the stretch reflex, you need to hold your stretch for about 30 seconds. Studies suggest that holding less than this makes stretches ineffective, while holding longer provides no added benefit.
- **Keep breathing.** Some people naturally tend to hold their breath while stretching, but breathing naturally keeps oxygen flowing to your muscles as you work them, and makes you feel more relaxed. (In yoga, breathing is an essential part of stretching.) Though breathing technique isn't critical with static stretching, some experts suggest exhaling as you move into your stretch, breathing normally as you hold, and inhaling as you return to your starting position.
- **Avoid bouncing.** Forget the quick, forceful stretches you learned in high school gym class: They're liable to make muscles extend beyond where they can safely go, which can cause tears like the kind you see in an overstretched rubber band—creating more stiffness, not less.
- **Don't cheat.** You'll be tempted to contort your body or use other muscles to compensate for stiffness, especially if you're afraid of triggering pain, but maintaining proper form is essential for restoring normal movement.
- **Stop if it hurts.** If you hurt, ask your physical therapist for other suggestions on working toward your goals, or check with your doctor about adjusting your pain medication.

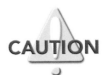

CAUTION

The American Physical Therapy Association says it's essential to consult a physical therapist before attempting any stretching exercises if you have pain other than simple stiffness or soreness anywhere in your body. (Ditto if you suffer from a medical condition or have a history of health trouble.) Even if you're exercising with a PT's okay, stop stretching immediately if you feel dizzy or experience any pain, instability, tingling, or numbness.

Fundamental Flexes

There are dozens of different stretches that might help your particular pain or condition; your physical therapist can help you choose the best ones for you. The following easy exercises provide a basic program that hits major muscle groups without putting undue strain on any part of the body.

To start your program, consider stretching every other day. As exercises become easier, you can start stretching every day. For best results, do each stretch at least four times, but stop if you feel overly uncomfortable or notice any pain.

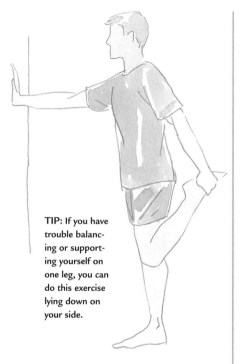

TIP: If you have trouble balancing or supporting yourself on one leg, you can do this exercise lying down on your side.

Quad Stretch

Targets front thigh (quadriceps) and hip muscles used for walking, running, and getting up and down from a chair.

1. With your left hand placed against a wall or chair for balance, bend your right knee and grasp your right ankle with your right hand, keeping your left knee slightly bent as it bears the weight of your body.

2. Gently pull your right foot toward your buttocks, stretching the muscles across the front of your thigh, keeping your upper leg straight. Hold your stomach in and keep your back straight.

3. Hold and repeat with the other leg.

Hamstring Stretch

Targets the back of the upper leg, where muscles are especially prone to injury.

1. Sit on an exercise bench (or a low table) with your right leg extended on the bench and your left foot flat on the floor with your left knee bent.

2. Resting your left hand on your right thigh, slowly slide your right fingers toward your toes without bending your right knee, keeping your back straight as you bend from the hip.

3. Hold and repeat with other leg.

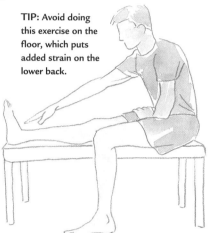

TIP: Avoid doing this exercise on the floor, which puts added strain on the lower back.

Seated Low-Back Stretch

Targets the muscles of the lower back, buttocks, and shoulders in an exercise that combines stretching and relaxation.

1. Sit all the way back in an armless straight-back chair with your feet together flat on the floor and your arms at your side.

2. Exhaling, lean forward from the waist so that your head rests on your knees and your hands and arms dangle to the floor.

3. Hold, breathing evenly as you let your back and shoulders completely relax.

4. Raise yourself slowly back to the starting position.

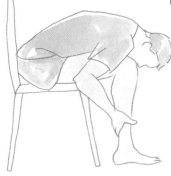

TIP: If your lower back is flexible enough, you can get an extra stretch by spreading your legs slightly and letting your head fall between your knees.

Hip Flexor Stretch

Hits mid-body muscles that support the torso and bear additional weight when you carry things.

1. Lie on your back with your knees bent and both feet flat on the floor about shoulder-width apart.

2. With the small of your back pressed toward the floor, bring your right knee toward your chest, pulling the upper leg back with both hands in the crook of your leg under your thigh.

3. Without arching your back, slowly extend your left leg along the floor.

4. Hold. Slowly return both legs to the starting position and repeat on the other side.

TIP: To maintain proper alignment, keep your neck straight and the small of your back pressed against the floor.

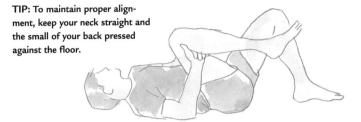

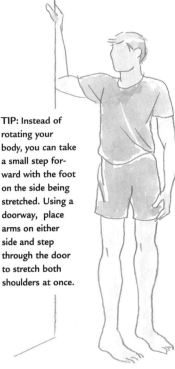

TIP: Instead of rotating your body, you can take a small step forward with the foot on the side being stretched. Using a doorway, place arms on either side and step through the door to stretch both shoulders at once.

Neck Stretch

Targets neck muscles prone to tension from supporting the head.

1. For a starting position, sit up straight in a sturdy armchair, facing forward with your arms on the armrests and shoulders relaxed.

2. Slowly turn your head to the right as far as it will comfortably go. Hold.

3. Slowly turn your head to left as far as it will comfortably go. Hold.

4. Slowly return to the starting position. Keeping your upper body straight, let your chin slowly drop toward your chest until you feel a slight tug at the back of your neck. Hold and slowly return to the starting position.

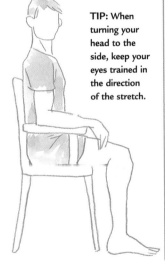

TIP: When turning your head to the side, keep your eyes trained in the direction of the stretch.

Wall Stretch

Targets the chest and shoulder muscles, improving flexibility for swinging motions.

1. Stand in a doorframe or at the end of a wall, feet shoulder-width apart.

2. Place your right forearm vertically against the wall with your elbow bent and your upper arm parallel to floor.

3. Keeping your lower arm steady against the wall, slowly rotate your body away from the wall and toward the opposite shoulder.

4. Hold and repeat with the left arm.

Behind-the-Back Stretch

Stretches triceps at the back of the upper arm, chest, and shoulders.

1. While standing or sitting in an upright position, bend your right arm behind your head so your right hand is directed toward the middle of your upper back and your right elbow is pointed upward.

2. Keeping your back straight, grasp your right elbow with your left hand and pull gently back and down until you feel a slight stretch along the back of your upper arm.

3. Hold, then repeat with the other arm.

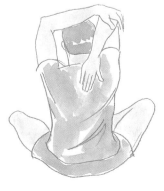

TIP: To make this stretch easier, don't pull on your elbow with the opposite hand, but rest your raised elbow against a doorjamb, moving your body closer to the doorjamb to push your upper arm to a vertical position.

Putting the Moves On

Some movement and posture therapies cross the line into what's usually considered alternative medicine—mainly because they combine physical disciplines with specific philosophies or Eastern spiritual practices. Doctors can't always back up the beliefs behind these therapies, but often recommend them anyway because many patients find the exercises helpful.

Few of these therapies have been thoroughly studied, though most of them have been used for years, if not centuries. Ask your physical therapist if any of the approaches below would be right for you, but be aware that PTs usually don't have the training to provide specialized therapies themselves. As a result, the cost of movement and posture therapies, which are seldom reimbursed by insurance, will probably come out of your own pocket. Are they worth it? You need to weigh the cost against the promised benefits.

YOGA: MELDING MIND AND MOVEMENT

Yoga is probably the most familiar movement therapy, and one of the oldest: It's thought to have been practiced in India for five thousand years. First introduced in the West during the 19th century, yoga did not gain mass appeal until the 1960s, but some of its ideas have become part of popular culture: If you have ever used

CAT ON YOUR BACK

Physical therapists often recommend the cat stretch, a simple yoga pose, to relieve lower back pain:

✸ Get down on the floor on your hands and knees, with your head and neck aligned and straight.

✸ Breathing in, arch your back slightly and look up so your eyes face forward, gently stretching your spine from your neck to your tailbone. Hold.

✸ Breathing out, lower your head and pull up on your stomach, rounding your back. Tuck your chin toward your chest and hold, breathing evenly.

✸ Slowly return to the starting position and repeat.

Tip: You can also do the arching and rounding movements as separate exercises.

the terms "karma" or "centering," you've been influenced by yoga.

For true believers, yoga is a rich and complex way of life meant to lead toward enlightenment through a series of stages that address everything from ethics to eating habits and personal hygiene. Along the way, practitioners learn exercise, breathing and meditation techniques to foster "oneness" between body and mind. (The word "yoga" comes from the Sanskrit word for union.)

Of the many different types of yoga, the most popular form in the West is hatha yoga, which combines breathing and physical poses known as asanas to influence the flow of "life energy" through a system of 72,000 channels said to flow throughout the body. According to the American Yoga Association, yoga exercises make your body stronger and more flexible while improving circulation and activating endorphins—feel-good chemicals that can help minimize pain. At the same time, breathing and meditation are said to calm the mind, reduce stress, and boost energy.

THE BOTTOM LINE: Whether yoga can affect brain chemicals or get your body coursing with life energy is open to debate, but using breathing to reduce tension and stretching exercises to promote strength and resilience is within the bounds of accepted medical practice. For example, one British study from the mid-1990s found that yoga therapy could benefit people with rheumatoid arthritis.

T'AI CHI: ACTION AND ENERGY

Technically, t'ai chi is a martial art, but you won't be breaking bricks (or heads). Instead, this Chinese movement therapy (more accurately called t'ai chi ch'uan) combines breathing with slow sequences of graceful movements. Like yoga, it's meant to promote the flow of energy through a system of meridians, promote tranquillity, and unite the mind, body, and spirit.

Though it's a part of traditional Chinese medicine, t'ai chi isn't meant to cure, but to prevent health problems that can lead to pain by making you stronger both inside and out. Proponents say it makes you more flexible, improves circulation, promotes balance and coordination, and enhances your overall sense of well-being.

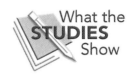

What the **STUDIES** Show

A recent study presented to the American Psychiatric Association supports claims that yoga can help relieve chronic pain. UCLA researchers asked 18 volunteers suffering from ailments like migraines and osteoarthritis to participate in 90-minute yoga sessions three times a week. After a month of doing exercises that released physical tension, most said their pain had eased to the point where they needed less pain medication from their doctors.

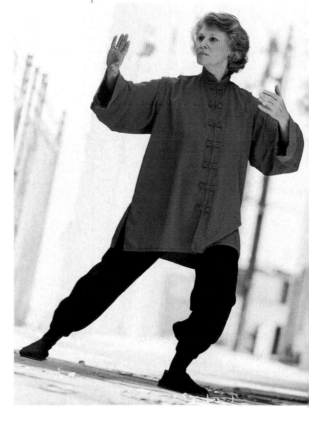

97

LEARNING MOVEMENT METHODS

You can pick up movement therapies like yoga and t'ai chi from books and videos, but it's better to learn from a teacher who can assess your condition and give you pointers on proper technique.

To find an instructor, check the yellow pages under "yoga." Some yoga centers also offer t'ai chi.

Classes generally have between 5 and 20 students and last about an hour. Wear comfortable clothing and don't be surprised if you're asked to take off your shoes and socks. The class should start with gentle warm-ups and easy moves if you're inexperienced, and the atmosphere should be relaxed but focused. Don't take on poses that feel uncomfortable or complex, and don't push yourself too hard—part of the joy is learning, practicing, and improving over time. Once you've learned some basic moves, start practicing at home, preferably every day.

Millions of people in China perform t'ai chi daily to calm the mind and stimulate self-healing. These veterans make t'ai chi look easy, but properly executing movements in smooth sequences (lasting anywhere from five to 40 minutes) takes concentration, control, and practice.

THE BOTTOM LINE: As with yoga, it's reasonable to believe that moving the body, breathing deeply, and concentrating your mind can help improve range of motion, keep you strong, distract you from pain, and improve your mood. For example, in one study of 120 experienced Chinese t'ai chi "players" (as they're known), more than 90 percent said they felt more cheerful and optimistic after practicing. In the West, studies suggest that t'ai chi improves breathing and reduces symptoms of stress.

THE ALEXANDER TECHNIQUE: POLICING YOUR POSTURE

In the late 1800s, an Australian actor named Frederick Matthias Alexander found himself in a quandary: Performing was making him lose his voice. Watching himself practice in front of a mirror, he concluded that his tense and unnatural posture while speaking was the cause. When he corrected his posture, his voice returned to normal: Voilà! After publishing his method in 1908, he gained a wide following, especially among people in the performing arts, and the Alexander Technique is now taught by thousands of trained specialists worldwide.

You don't have to practice stagecraft to benefit: Physical therapists in principle agree with Alexander's notion that poor posture habits like cradling a phone with your shoulder or hunching over a computer keyboard can cause tension and pain. More subtly, the Alexander Technique teaches that you need a balanced relationship between your head, neck, and spine. In fact, according to the technique's adherents, many people in pain (or at risk for it) need to relearn basic movements such as sitting and standing.

The Alexander Technique isn't so much therapy as instruction, usually in one-on-one sessions. Your teacher guides your body into more natural positions while explaining how to be more aware of the way you hold your body throughout the day.

THE BOTTOM LINE: The basic ideas behind the Alexander Technique appear to be sound, especially when treating chronic neck and back problems or pain from repetitive motion. (Many musicians and performers still swear by it.) A British medical journal noted a study in which patients at one pain clinic said the Alexander Technique was the best of 13 activities tried during a pain management course. Still, Alexander himself was wary of overanalyzing his technique for fear it would be misunderstood, and few researchers have studied it.

Hands-On Healing

If you want to change the kinks and quirks of your posture and movement, there are two ways to go about it. One is to learn new motions through movement therapy. The other is to have someone else move your body for you—through touch and manipulation therapies such as massage and chiropractic.

As with movement therapies, these hands-on methods aren't always considered part of conventional medicine, and a primary care physician may not think to recommend them. But physical therapists, pain specialists, and rehabilitation doctors often embrace them for certain types of pain because many sufferers say they work—and research, though not as conclusive as doctors would like, tends to back up satisfied patients.

MASSAGE: THE ULTIMATE FEEL-GOOD THERAPY

It's hard to argue with the "mmm-good" feeling you get from a massage, and the commonsense notion that rubbing and pressing can ease pain has been a staple of care and comfort around the world for centuries. In ancient Greece and Rome, physicians such as Hippocrates considered massage the main treatment for pain.

Today there are many different forms of massage, but the most popular in the West is known as Swedish massage, a system of techniques grounded in anatomy that was pioneered by a 19th-century gymnast named Per Henrik Ling. Massage therapists using his methods say that stroking, kneading, rubbing, and hacking can relax tight muscles, limber up stiff joints, boost circulation, clear the body of wastes, and trigger the release of painkilling endorphins.

Not all of these claims hold up under scrutiny. For example, studies suggest massage actually doesn't boost blood flow to muscles. But other research finds massage has a wide range of effects such as boosting the immune system, lowering blood sugar in diabetic children, and improving mood—even in people who give massages rather than receive them.

DIFFERENT STROKES

Whether you're laying on your own hands or treating yourself to a session with a professional, look to a handful of basic techniques to make the most of a massage:

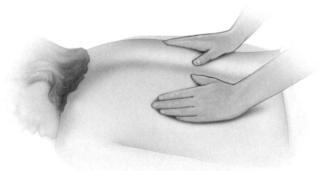

Kneading
Technical name: petrissage. A rhythmic squeezing and releasing of muscles with alternate hands to stretch and relax muscles, particularly in fleshy areas such as the thighs.

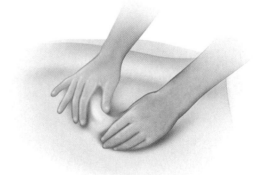

Stroking
Technical name: effleurage. A gentle, gliding action in which hands move rhythmically over the skin in a circular or fanning pattern. Ideal for stimulating circulation and relaxing tense muscles.

The public image of massage has suffered over the years as seedy "massage parlors" have sometimes been fronts for prostitution, but on-the-level massage therapists have helped restore legitimacy to their profession in part by establishing professional standards. Look for therapists who have been certified or accepted as members by groups such as the National Certification Board for Therapeutic Massage and Bodywork or the American Massage Therapy Association.

THE BOTTOM LINE: Whatever its proven effects, there's little doubt massage makes you feel relaxed, eases tension, and promotes feelings of well-being. And there's reason to believe it helps with pain. For example, in one study of 13 people with soft-tissue injuries, a few minutes of friction massage relieved pain for periods ranging from 20 seconds to 48 hours. You have little to lose: Even a nonprofessional, no-cost self-massage or a rubdown from a loved one can help ease pain and lift your spirits.

MANIPULATION: GETTING THE SPINE IN LINE

Being "manipulated" sounds unsavory, but in this case, the term refers to the pressing, thrusting, or twisting of the body to ease pain and improve health. Its basic techniques are practiced by

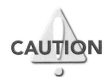

CAUTION

Manipulation involves applying forceful pressure, which raises a small risk of serious injury such as stroke or paralysis, especially when it involves the neck. Check with your doctor before undergoing manipulation, and avoid procedures involving the neck if you have arthritis or ankylosing spondylitis, a chronic inflammation of the spine. Also be wary of manipulation if your spinal cord is being compressed by a disk, arthritis, or a tumor.

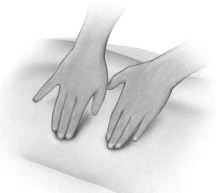

Friction
Technical name: frottage. Deep, penetrating, steady pressure on a single point, or in a circular pattern in a small area, usually applied with three fingers or the thumbs. Particularly good for releasing tension around the shoulders and spine.

Hacking
Technical name: tapotement. A brisk, drumming action using the sides of the hands to deliver sharp taps to fleshy, muscular areas.

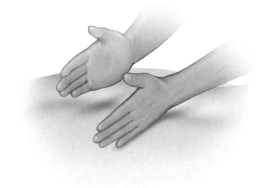

ELECTRIFICATION PROJECT

Using a combination of high-tech gizmo and benign physical stimulation, some pain sufferers find relief through a treatment known as TENS—transcutaneous electrical nerve stimulation.

Patients wear a portable pager-like device containing a battery that sends low-level electrical impulses into the skin through wires attached to the body by electrodes.

The treatment is controversial because doctors don't understand how it works—or even whether electrodes are best placed where you hurt or away from the site of pain. One theory is that the gentle TENS tingling distracts people from pain, while another theory holds that the electricity closes the gate on the pain pathway through the nervous system. TENS also appears to relax muscles and trigger the release of endorphins. Some believe that whatever relief patients feel is entirely placebo effect—consistent with its providing relief of intractable pain in about 30 percent of cases.

Studies on TENS's effectiveness have produced mixed results. But many people choose to try it anyway, because the treatment is safe and seems to help some patients.

physical therapists, osteopaths, and especially chiropractors, who concentrate on manipulating the spine.

Manipulation is hugely popular: Chiropractors are the third-largest group of healthcare professionals in the U.S., after physicians and dentists. But the value of chiropractic treatment has long been controversial. In the 1960s, the American Medical Association dismissed chiropractic as an "unscientific cult." It's partly a war of ideas: Chiropractors hold that correctable misalignments in the spine known as subluxations not only cause back pain, but trigger problems throughout the entire body—an unproven theory that many doctors don't accept. Osteopaths, who (unlike chiropractors) earn the equivalent of a medical degree, don't speak of subluxations, but say correcting mechanical defects in joints, muscles, ligaments, and connective tissue can ease pain and strain, and promote better overall health.

Whatever the underlying ideas, recent research suggests that manipulation is useful for treating low-back and neck pain. In fact, the U.S. Department of Health and Human Services now officially recognizes spinal manipulation as a viable treatment for low-back pain—the main reason people see chiropractors.

THE BOTTOM LINE: Spinal manipulation can help relieve low-back pain, though the strongest evidence is in acute pain lasting three weeks or less. It's less clear how valuable manipulation is for longer-lasting back pain or conditions such as osteoarthritis.

MIXED METHODS

A number of "bodywork" therapies combine different elements of physical therapy, movement/posture therapy, massage, and manipulation. Among them:

Rolfing. Also known as structural integration, this therapy was developed by an American biochemist named Ida Rolf after an osteopath's treatment of her displaced rib sparked her interest in manipulation. Like spinal manipulators, she believed function improves when body parts are properly aligned. However, her method involves stretching and loosening the sinewy connective tissue surrounding muscles by applying firm pressure with knuckles, fingers and elbows.

Hellerwork. Joseph Heller, an engineer who worked with Rolf, developed this approach by combining elements of Rolfing with "movement re-education" that teaches stress-free ways to go about daily actions. Heller's method also involves dialogue therapy in which patients talk about emotions triggered by the release of tension in the body.

Tragerwork. Also called "psychophysical integration," this method was developed by a doctor named Milton Trager, who was influenced by his knowledge of transcendental meditation. Tragerwork therapists use light, gentle, repetitive movements such as rocking, stretching, and jiggling to induce a meditative state that encourages patients to give up control of their muscles.

The Exercise Effect

If you don't feel like exercising, no one can blame you. After all, even people who aren't dealing with pain have trouble getting their bodies into action. At least one-quarter of American adults are totally inactive—and that number exceeds one-third for people over age 55. But the flip side is that at least two-thirds of your peers get some physical activity—and you'll be best off if you're among them.

"Bed rest is seldom recommended anymore, even for people experiencing pain," says Dr. Materson of the University of Texas Medical School and Baylor College of Medicine. It's easy to see why when you tally the cost of being immobile. One landmark study of healthy young men found that three weeks of bed rest cut their maximal oxygen uptake (a basic measure of cardiovascular fitness) by 27 percent—and some elements of cardiovascular function started to nosedive

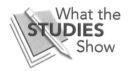
What the STUDIES Show

In a study of 60 people with the generalized pain condition called fibromyalgia, researchers broke participants into three groups. Two groups took part in aerobic exercise or stress management, while a third acted as a control group for comparison. After 14 weeks, both treatment groups had less pain and disability than the control group—but the aerobics group did best of all.

within two days. Other research shows that bed rest reduces strength by as much as 1 percent a day, decreases the ability of bones and ligaments to bear weight, restricts range of motion, and hinders coordination.

But if pain has you sidelined, there's a brightly glimmering silver lining:

Whatever you lose from being inactive, you can gain back with regular exercise. And the sooner you start, the better. Your program might be different than the next person's, but no matter what you choose to do, physical activity not only can ease pain and restore function over the long term, it tends to relieve fear of movement.

Just as vital, exercise provides a sense of control over your life—important because if you feel self-empowered, studies suggest you're more likely to lead a richer, fuller life despite pain.

AEROBICS: OPEN YOUR HEART

Anyone who doubts that staying fit improves overall function and fends off disability can find proof in older people who keep active as they age. Studies find that regular aerobic exercise—even if you start as an adult—can extend "functional independence" by 10 to 20 years!

Aerobics are what most people imagine when they think of exercise—walking, running, bicycling, swimming, rowing, skiing, or any other activity that raises your heart rate and makes you breathe harder for a sustained period of time. When you exercise aerobically, you work big muscle groups that need lots of oxygen to keep going ("aerobic" means "with oxygen"), boosting demands on the heart and lungs. As these organs become stronger, your entire body benefits. Regular aerobic exercise reduces risk of often painful diseases such as heart disease and diabetes; helps control weight, which eases strain on muscles and bones; and reduces risks of certain forms of cancer. Aerobic activity also triggers the release of endorphins (the body's natural painkillers), relieves depression, helps you sleep better, and promotes feelings of well-being.

The general rule for improving aerobic conditioning is to exercise hard enough to make your heart beat at between 60 and 80 percent of the maximal rate for your age. But don't worry about the math: If you're breaking a sweat and feel slightly short of breath but can still comfortably carry on a conversation while exercising, you're probably at the right intensity level. At first, you'll want to exercise lightly, but as you become more fit, you can start pushing yourself harder, depending on your age, overall health, fitness level, and goals. Strive to work out at least three to five days a week, and to exercise for at least 20 minutes each time you work out.

MOVING TOWARD MOTION

The first step is often the toughest one to take. But increasing your physical activity doesn't have to be discouragingly difficult if you bear these points in mind:

▶ **Take it easy.** Terms like "workout" and "regimen" can sound daunting, but don't lose heart before you start: Exercise doesn't have to be vigorous to do you good. In fact, studies find that moderate—not to mention fun—activities such as bowling, golf, gardening, and walking deliver many of the same health benefits as high-powered exercise. Can you manage half an hour of physical fun several times a week? If so, you've just met the health-improvement standards recommended by the U.S. Centers for Disease Control and Prevention and the American College of Sports Medicine.

▶ **Break it up.** There's no need for the half-hour mark to be a stumbling block, either. If you can't manage 30 minutes of steady activity (or just don't have the time), studies find you can break exercise into shorter segments spread throughout the day—say, three 10-minute walks—to get many of the same benefits you'd receive from a longer workout.

▶ **Check with the authorities.** Before you start any regular program, get an okay from your doctor to make sure it's appropriate for you. Your pain is only one consideration: If you're over 40, you should also be evaluated for heart disease risk factors, including high blood pressure.

▶ **Keep it real.** If you're working with a physical therapist, follow the PT's recommendations to make sure you have realistic goals and are pacing yourself properly. Start by doing less than you think you can and gradually increase the physical demands you place on yourself. It's common for beginning exercisers to overdo it at the outset, which may increase your pain and discourage you from continuing to exercise.

GETTING STRONG NOW

If pain makes you constantly feel like an underdog, it's time to make like Sylvester Stallone's stalwart Rocky. But remember that you don't have to get yourself into fighting trim. All that's necessary to build muscle power is that you demand a little more of your muscles than they're used to. That's the idea behind strength training, in which you exert your muscles against some form of resistance, which can be provided by free weights, exercise machines, elastic bands, your own body weight—or even a stationary object like a wall.

Strength training isn't just for the spandex-and-mirrors crowd. Studies of older people, who—like many victims of pain—tend to lose strength from inactivity, find that even 80- and 90-year-olds can make their legs twice as strong with just two months of resistance exercises.

Unlike aerobic exercise, which conditions the whole body at once, strength exercises target isolated muscles or muscle groups, one at a time. But that doesn't mean that a workout takes forever to complete. You can tone up the major muscle groups in the chest, arms, abdomen, back, shoulders, and legs with as few as six exercises.

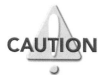

CAUTION

If a resistance exercise causes pain or makes you feel uncomfortable, stop doing it—you may be using too much weight or improper form. If you're already experiencing pain before an exercise, don't lift through the pain. Instead, ask your physical therapist how to perform the exercise through a limited range of motion. That way, you can avoid the pain, but still gain significant benefit from the part of the lift that you do.

- ▶ A typical workout using weights or resistance machines like those you find in a gym is built around several key principles. First, lift weight that's heavy enough to make your muscles too tired to go on after 8 to 12 repetitions. This breaks muscle tissue down and causes it to rebuild even stronger.
- ▶ When lifting becomes easy after 12 repetitions, you can add slightly more weight to keep muscles challenged. It's not necessary to do more than one set of repetitions, which produces little added strength but increases your risk of injury, especially if you're just starting out. (If you do multiple sets, be sure to rest one to three minutes between sets.)
- ▶ Most important, perform exercises with good form, moving the weight slowly and smoothly through a muscle's full range of motion.

A Road to Recovery

Driving on a winding, two-lane country road outside Lafayette, Indiana, Marc Brown suffered a head-on crash with a semi around a curve. He spent more than 11 months in the hospital and had 41 different operations to repair the damage—including broken bones in both legs, a shattered hip, an arm that was almost torn off, internal injuries that left him with only half his stomach, and burns that required skin grafts. "I was like the Six Million Dollar Man," he says. "They had to put me back together again."

The accident more than 30 years ago changed Brown's life. He has spent decades working on rehabilitation while also dealing with pain. "As it was, the doctors didn't think I'd ever walk again." The key to proving them wrong, he soon realized, was physical therapy. "Physical therapy not only mends the body, it keeps your mind functioning and keeps you hopeful that you'll get back on your feet again," he says. "Physical therapists are great. They understand sometimes better than doctors what's going to help your body and ease your pain. They know you can do it. But it's up to you to deliver."

It's been a slow road. "I'd sometimes become complacent, so every few years I'd get new exercises or a new physical therapist to keep me moving ahead." He especially remembers working on excruciating but necessary exercises in which he would try to bend his leg with weighted ankles to regain function in his knee.

The effort has paid off. In 1990 he started getting out of his wheelchair. "I really started regaining function around 1995," he says. A breakthrough, however, came just two years ago, when Brown started taking a COX-2 nonsteroidal anti-inflammatory medication. By significantly reducing the pain in his body, Brown has been able to concentrate even more on his fitness: "It's been a godsend. If I'd had that drug 10 years ago, I'd be even further ahead."

Today Brown works out at least once a day—walking, range-of-motion exercises, light weightlifting, and going up and down steps. "I've got a whole sheet of things I do," he says. He also lowers himself into a Jacuzzi before and after exercising. "It takes a lot of the pain away. "The water loosens tight muscles and makes moving easier—plus, it just makes me feel good."

Thanks to this mix of one medication and physical therapy, Brown can now walk without a cane. Managing his pain and regaining function have let him concentrate on a project he loves: FosterCare Luggage for Kids, an Indianapolis-based organization he founded to provide proper suitcases to foster children when they move.

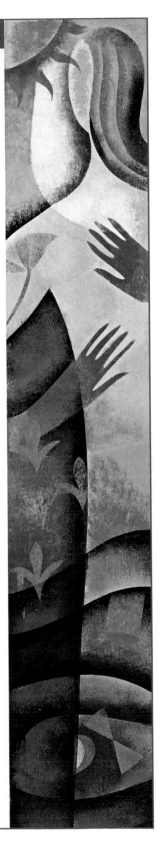

5

ALTERNATIVE APPROACHES

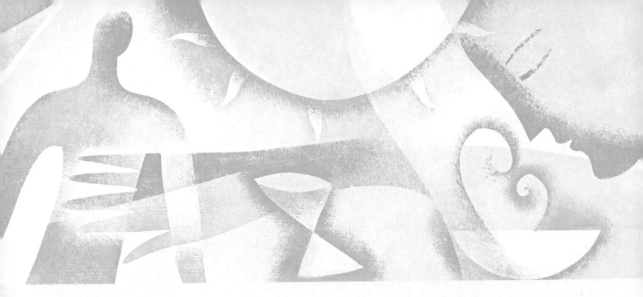

Western medicine, based on scientific research, has long been skeptical of many alternative forms of treating the sick, such as acupuncture and hypnosis, that do not meet the strict criteria of rational proof required by science. In the field of pain management, however, doctors have seen patients receive relief from some of these practices that they have not received from other forms of treatment. When side effects are minimal, doctors are beginning to look more kindly on such helpful alternatives that complement the use of drug and exercise therapies.

Time was, alternative treatments were strictly seen as fringe medicine. The feeling among most doctors (and many patients) was that therapies outside the corral of traditional Western medicine were unsound, unproven, unscientific, and, in some cases, potentially unsafe. These criticisms haven't gone away, and warrant serious consideration. But as the popularity of unconventional treatments has exploded in recent years, alternative medicine has moved away from the fringes and closer to the mainstream.

For patients, it's easy to see why. "Alternative" medicine offers just what it suggests: another approach. Western treatments tend to be expensive, doctor-directed, technological (relying mainly on drugs and surgery), and narrowly focused. "Physicians are accustomed to dividing up the body in their minds," says Joseph Audette, M.D., clinical director of the Integrative Care Clinic at Harvard Medical School. "If you have pain in your right hip, you only look at what's happening there, not in the leg, the head, the neck, or anywhere else. But that approach often doesn't work, especially with chronic conditions, and particularly with pain."

Alternatives and Chronic Pain

Alternative treatments, in contrast to traditional medicine, tend to be relatively cheap (though out-of-pocket costs can add up), patient-controlled, and low-tech. Just as important, they tend to see the body—along with the mind and, often, the spirit—as an integrated whole, not as a collection of isolated parts.

What treatments are "alternative"? Start with many of the therapies already discussed in this book—therapies that pain specialists often consider valuable ways to manage suffering. These treatments include:

- **Mental techniques** such as distraction, visualization, meditation, and hypnosis
- **Therapies involving pleasant diversions** such as music and laughter

- **Relaxation regimens** such as deep breathing, progressive muscle relaxation, and biofeedback
- **Healing-touch techniques** including massage, manipulation, and even (in some doctors' minds) certain elements of physical therapy
- **Movement and stretching disciplines** like yoga and t'ai chi
- **Posture-correcting and bodywork methods** such as the Alexander Technique, Hellerwork, and Rolfing

Other techniques sometimes used to relieve pain include acupuncture, aromatherapy, homeopathy, magnet therapy, and herbal medicine.

Nobody should rely on any of these therapies alone or consider them a substitute for medical care from a doctor. But some doctors are becoming more open to making such treatments an adjunct to traditional medicine—substituting the word "complementary" for "alternative." In fact, surveys show that as many as 60 percent of doctors have recommended complementary alternative medicine, or CAM, to their patients.

Why are some physicians bringing CAM in from the cold? "Those of us who treat chronic pain often don't feel we have a lot to offer patients with traditional Western medicine, or we may have concerns about serious side effects or the addictive properties of certain drugs," says Audette. "As a result, I think we reach out to alternative therapies even more than other doctors, and listen when patients tell us they work." Furthermore, clinical experience and a limited—but growing—amount of research suggests that some alternative methods may be scientifically justified, though none have been conclusively proved.

QUESTIONS AND CONCERNS

The public has led the drive for greater acceptance of alternative therapies. Still, many patients are reluctant to go outside traditional channels for care even when doctors suggest it might help. "People tend to be of two minds," says Audette. "Some are fearful of going into the community for care because, let's face it, you generally don't get these treatments from established hospitals. Other people are so frustrated by what they've been through with traditional medicine that they jump at the chance to try something different, even though they often have an idealized notion of what alternative therapies can do."

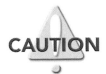

The best approach lies somewhere in between. Using alternative therapies raises a number of issues that you should consider when deciding if a treatment is right for you.

■ **Safety.** Few alternative therapies have been subjected to the kind of rigorous scientific study that's standard for treatments embraced by conventional medicine. As a result, the risks of alternative therapies are often poorly understood. For some types of therapies—particularly herbal remedies whose potency can sometimes rival that of drugs—this can be a serious concern, especially if you use them for long periods or are taking other medications. But many alternative therapies, such as massage and mind/body methods, are innocuous. "One of the appeals of alternative therapies is that, for the most part, they're safe," says Audette, "especially when compared with the risks of most medical treatments for pain."

■ **Effectiveness.** What little research has been done on alternative therapies is often (but not always) poorly designed, so there's a general lack of scientific evidence that they really work. Instead, alternative advocates tend to invoke testimonials (useful information, but far from conclusive) or will cite a long history of use going back decades, centuries, or even millennia. Skeptics contend that benefits credited to alternative therapies are really just placebo effect. Barring placebo-controlled studies, there may be little reason to think otherwise.

■ **Quality.** Practitioners of alternative therapies such as chiropractic, acupuncture, massage, and various forms of bodywork often are certified by professional organizations and, in some cases, licensed by their state. Naturally, competence and effectiveness can vary. However, some forms of therapy lack any kind of oversight whatsoever. Case in point: Because herbal and nutritional remedies are classified as supplements rather than medicines, the Food and Drug Administration doesn't regulate them. That means you need to take manufacturers' word that they're filling bottles with what they say they are and that the product is of therapeutic potency.

THE BOTTOM LINE: "A lot of alternative medicine is done with a certain amount of ignorance," says Audette. "We simply don't

ALTERNATIVE BANDWAGON

In 1993 the National Institutes of Health established the National Center for Complementary and Alternative Medicine to build a base of research on what was already an exploding field. In the decade that followed, use of alternative medicine has continued to grow:

> Through the end of the 1990s, visits to doctors held steady, but visits to alternative therapists boomed by 47 percent.

> By the late 1990s, the number of visits to alternative practitioners exceeded visits to primary-care physicians.

> In 1998 *The Journal of the American Medical Association* reported that during a single year, more than 40 percent of Americans had used at least one alternative therapy.

> Americans spend more than $20 billion a year on alternative treatments.

know well enough how to set up a treatment plan based on research, so it can be hit or miss." Use your common sense and discuss the options with friends and family, as well as your doctor. Weigh the costs (unlikely to be reimbursed by insurers) against the supposed benefits. Then give it a try and see if it helps. Don't be surprised if a given treatment doesn't work. And don't put all your hope into a single therapy. "The best results usually come from combinations of therapies," says Audette. "One therapy, such as acupuncture, might calm pain signals, while another, such as bodywork, may correct the cause of the pain." And, again, any alternative treatments should only be in addition to regular medical treatment.

The Point of Acupuncture

It seems counterintuitive to ease pain by having someone stick needles in your skin. But that's the promise of acupuncture, a treatment that's been part of traditional Chinese medicine for more than 2,000 years. Though it's said to alleviate a variety of health problems, one of its most common (and scientifically credible) uses in the U.S. is relieving pain, including backaches, migraine headaches, and fibromyalgia.

The idea behind acupuncture is that health depends upon the movement of *qi* (pronounced "chee"), a vital life force believed to travel the body through a system of channels, or meridians. Pain or disease occurs when the flow of *qi* becomes blocked or imbalanced. Placing needles at specific points along the meridians is thought to restore proper energy flow, establishing balance, healing the body, and easing pain.

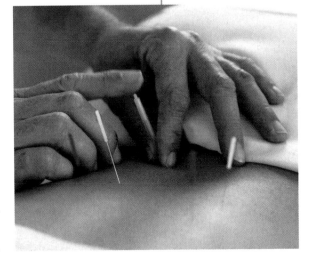

Though known in America since the 1820s, acupuncture's popularity took off after President Richard Nixon visited China in 1972. But many Western doctors remain skeptical about acupuncture, saying it has no rational basis because the meridian system doesn't correspond to any feature of the anatomy (and no one has found any *qi*).

As researchers have studied acupuncture in recent years, however, they've made a number of intriguing discoveries. For example, acupuncture points are often near major nerve endings, and the skin at those points has been shown to conduct electricity differently than other areas of the body. There's substantial evidence that acupuncture triggers the release of natural painkillers such as endorphins and an amino acid derivative known as 5-HTP, which is thought to ease migraine pain. Other research suggests that acupuncture can alter immune function and cause changes in the brain detectable with new imaging technology.

By the late 1990s, acupuncture had gained credibility in the medical community, although much still needs to be learned. For example, after reviewing hundreds of studies, a National Institutes of Health consensus panel concluded in 1997 that strong evidence supports acupuncture's use for dental pain, menstrual cramps, tennis elbow, fibromyalgia, and a variety of other conditions. Less strong—but still promising—evidence also suggests that acupuncture may be a useful adjunct treatment for headache, myofascial pain, osteoarthritis, low-back pain, and carpal tunnel syndrome. In some cases, the panel noted, the evidence supporting acupuncture was as strong as data backing conventional medical treatments—but acupuncture had far fewer unpleasant side effects. At about the same time, the Food and Drug Administration (FDA) approved acupuncture needles as bona fide medical devices on a par with scalpels and syringes.

THE BOTTOM LINE: It still isn't entirely clear how acupuncture works, but studies (and many doctors' clinical experience) suggest it can help with a variety of pains, along with various pain-causing conditions. While still mainly practiced by non-physicians, a number of medical schools across the country (including Harvard) now offer courses on acupuncture for physicians, and enough doctors have become practitioners that they've formed their own organization, the American Academy of Medical Acupuncture (800-521-2262 or www.medical-acupuncture.org). Still, acupuncture may not help everybody, and treatment costs (ranging from $35 to $150 per session) can add up. If you don't show improvement after six sessions, acupuncture may prove ineffective for you. Avoid acupuncture if you have a bleeding disorder or take anticoagulant medication. And if you have a pacemaker, don't get treatments in which needles are electrified.

NEEDLE KNOWLEDGE: WHAT TO EXPECT

First things first: Does acupuncture hurt? When the needle is inserted, expect to feel a prick, tingling, or ache that quickly goes away. (Putting a positive spin on it, practitioners say this means they've accessed *qi* and have found the right spot.) After initial placement, the procedure may be entirely painless as needles are left in place for periods ranging from a few seconds to a few hours (15 to 30 minutes is typical), depending on your condition.

To learn more about your particular case, your practitioner will conduct an assessment that's arguably as important as the treatment itself. Different schools of acupuncture use different diagnostic methods (as well as treatment techniques). Typically, you'll be asked about your lifestyle, medical history, and diet, but practitioners also look at physical clues such as pallor. Don't be surprised if your tongue and ears get a careful look-see, and expect the practitioner to take your pulse in six different ways on each wrist—12 positions corresponding to the dozen major meridians. Some disciplines also rely on palpation of soft tissues, such as the abdomen.

Once needles are in, other techniques may be used. Often, practitioners twist or manipulate needles to regulate the flow of *qi*, which produces a dull ache known as *deqi*. This may feel uncomfortable, but some researchers speculate the *deqi* sensation is critical for chemicals to be released in the nervous system. Needles can also be heated using burners stoked with an herb known as moxa to conduct heat to the skin (moxibustion), or charged with a low-level electrical current (electroacupuncture). Often practitioners forgo needles altogether, heating acupoints by placing small, smoldering vessels called moxa cones on the body, or holding the hot end of a cigar-like moxa stick near the skin.

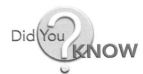

Did You **KNOW**

The World Health Organization lists more than 40 conditions for which acupuncture may offer relief, promote rehabilitation, or provide protection. In addition to pain, these include nausea, vomiting, and other gastrointestinal problems; addictions to alcohol, tobacco, and other drugs; asthma and bronchitis; and stroke.

PRESSURE TACTICS

Another no-needle way to stimulate the flow of *qi* in traditional Chinese medicine is putting pressure on acupoints using fingers, thumbs, or even feet or knees. Similar in principle to acupuncture, this form of massage, known as acupressure, probably predates the use of needles. A similar traditional therapy in Japan has evolved into the pressure-point massage technique known as shiatsu.

Using the Force

Acupuncture is far from the only alternative therapy whose practitioners invoke energy flow to explain its effects. In fact, much of alternative medicine falls back on "life force" concepts that seem vague and quasi-superstitious to Western doctors. But experience with acupuncture has suggested that seemingly irrational ideas may produce therapies that work—perhaps in some unknown or as-yet-undetectable way.

In the case of other energy-based therapies, the evidence for their effectiveness isn't necessarily better than (or even as good as) that for acupuncture, but they tend to be safer because they don't entail penetrating the skin. Many of these therapies—using varying philosophies that strike the healing energy theme—require nothing more threatening than the touch of a therapist's hands.

SHIATSU: PUTTING ON PRESSURE

Shiatsu is a massage therapy that comes from Japan but is based on the traditional Chinese concepts of energy flow and meridi-

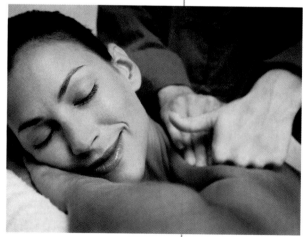

ans that underlie acupuncture. In fact, shiatsu (a word that means "finger pressure") is closely related to acupressure: Practitioners use hands and body weight (as well as stretching and squeezing techniques) to put pressure on specific points known as *tsubos*.

Though influenced by ancient therapies, shiatsu is actually fairly recent, developed during the 19th century by a Japanese practitioner who also drew on Western knowledge of anatomy and physiology. Some practitioners in the West prefer to explain shiatsu's relaxing and health-promoting effects in physiological terms, saying it regulates hormones, relaxes muscles, eliminates wastes, and boosts circulation.

Much of shiatsu focuses on diagnosis, using a method known as *hara*, in which energy is detected and mapped by palpating areas of the abdomen said to correspond to other sites in the body. Your therapist typically asks detailed questions and conducts a diagnostic exam before beginning treatment, which usually lasts about an hour and covers the entire body, often starting at a point just below the navel.

THE BOTTOM LINE: Shiatsu's specific methods and theories have not been scientifically proven or even studied to any great extent, so there's little evidence that it's effective against arthritis, headaches, menstrual pain, or any other condition it's often used to treat. Still, you may find it relaxing (though it has a reputation for being a "robust" therapy that may not always be comfortable), and it may work in ways similar to those shown for acupuncture.

THERAPEUTIC TOUCH: HEALING HANDS

Laying on of hands has been a staple of faith healers for thousands of years, but was brought into hospitals through the nursing profession during the 1970s. It isn't strictly a form of spiritual healing, however. Practitioners of therapeutic touch—sometimes called TT—say people have individual energy fields that interact with each other and affect the environment around them. What's more, therapists say they can ease pain, reduce anxiety, and transfer healing energy to another person, sometimes without any physical contact.

It's a meditative process: The practitioner tries to attune her energy field with yours by quietly focusing on you and moving her hands several inches over your body to detect disruptions in your field. The therapist may use sweeping motions to direct your energy and use visualization to focus on healing your pain.

Studies of therapeutic touch have produced mixed but intriguing results. One study of 60 headache patients, for example, seemed to suggest it's a sham: While 90 percent of those who got real TT felt relief, so did 80 percent of those treated by fakers. The catch: Those who got the real treatment had less pain and used less pain medication afterward. Other studies have had similar results. In one fascinating example, 44 patients who'd had biopsies on their arms were told to put their affected limb through a hole in the wall, where it would be monitored by a machine. Unknown to them, half of the patients actually got TT and half got no treatment at all. Result: Biopsy wounds on 12 of the 22 who received therapeutic touch were completely healed after 16 days, but none of the wounds had healed on those who weren't treated.

THE BOTTOM LINE: The medical establishment is skeptical about therapeutic touch, though nurses in some hospitals incorporate it in their healing practices. With suggestive research backing it up and no downsides, it's a harmless, though unproven, option for treating pain.

REFLEXOLOGY: A TREAT FOR THE FEET

Most people find foot massage deeply relaxing (assuming your feet aren't ticklish). But reflexology takes the feet a step further. According to theories that evolved from ancient practices in China and were refined in the West during the 19th and 20th centuries, the feet and hands are covered with "reflex points" that match specific areas of the body. For example, points along the side of the feet between the instep and the heel correlate with regions of the spine, while points under the toes tie with various parts of the head. Putting pressure on reflex points is said to ease pain, stimulate natural healing, and promote well-being in corresponding zones of the body.

A number of theories attempt to explain how reflexology might work, none of them scientifically proved. Reflexologists contend that their treatments break down accumulations of waste formed from uric acid and calcium that concentrate around reflex points. They say this boosts blood flow, flushes away toxins, and opens up energy channels to the affected regions. It's also possible that sensory nerves in the feet send signals to the brain that loop back to the targeted area.

THE BOTTOM LINE: There's no scientific evidence that reflexology does what it says, but it's often used for stress-related disorders, suggesting its benefits may largely be due to relaxation. There's no denying the feet are exquisitely sensitive, with more than 7,000 nerve endings in each foot, and some people find that stimulating the feet can produce pleasant sensations elsewhere in the body. However, while extraordinarily safe for most people, reflexology should be avoided if you've had a fracture or reconstructive surgery in your feet or hands (also treated sometimes) or on areas where the skin is broken or infected. Pregnant women should avoid reflexology that stimulates the uterine points.

Relief ▶**TIP**

Reaching for Reflex Points

It's undoubtedly more pleasant (and, practitioners say, more effective) to have a trained therapist stimulate your feet, but there's no reason you can't try to reap some of reflexology's benefits on your own. A sample technique: Work your thumb along the inside edge of your foot from your heel to the tip of your big toe—a massage that hits reflex points for several sections of the spine, and may cross sites for the neck and a variety of organs.

REIKI: CHANGING CHANNELS

As with therapeutic touch, practitioners of this healing method purport to channel a vital force, which they call *reiki*—a Japanese term combining the words for "universal" (*rei*) and "life energy" (*ki*). Reiki was developed in the 19th century by a Japanese monk who studied and reinterpreted what apparently were ancient practices from Tibetan Buddhism. Practitioners focus on themselves as much as you: They pass through three training stages in which they become attuned to techniques they believe are necessary to channel energy. They also maintain that treating you can help rebalance their own energy.

In a typical treatment, you lie on a treatment table (no clothing removal required) while the practitioner places his hands on or near 12 basic positions—four each over the head, torso, and back. The practitioner holds his hands at each position for several minutes to balance your body's "energy centers." But you don't always need to be this close: Practitioners claim they can also transfer healing energy over distances.

THE BOTTOM LINE: Few studies have been done on reiki, and the ideas behind it strike many doctors as exotic and far-fetched. But, like therapeutic touch, it appears to have few drawbacks and may be worth using if it provides comfort or relaxation.

Senses and Substances

While many alternative therapies require you to believe in mysterious energy fields, others base their claims on purported powers from medicinal substances. Scientists have difficulty explaining how some medicinal therapies work, but like other forms of alternative medicine, these treatments have a long history—and legions of adherents.

Sometimes referring to their methods as "natural healing," alternative practitioners play up the fact that their treatments are gentle, non-invasive, and have few side effects. Does lack of side effects mean lack of any effect? Many doctors would say so—or argue that effects are due to the placebo effect.

HOMEOPATHY: LESS IS MORE

One of the most popular of alternative therapies, homeopathy is a healing system based on the idea that "like cures like"—sometimes called the law of similars. Though the basic concepts of homeopathy date back to Hippocrates, the system was developed in the late 18th century by a German doctor, Samuel Hahnemann, who was dissatisfied with the medicine of his day. He believed, on the basis of experiments, that substances capable of producing certain symptoms can cure the same symptoms—if used in highly diluted amounts—by stimulating the body to heal itself.

Homeopaths contend that the more a substance is diluted, the more powerful it becomes—a concept known as "potentization." In fact, the healing substance in many homeopathic remedies can't even be detected. But even when no molecules of the medicine are present, homeopaths say the substance leaves a "message" that the body responds to.

Homeopaths use more than 2,000 different remedies for a wide range of conditions, including inflammation, headaches, neuralgia, and fibromyalgia. Most remedies are based on plants, many of them poisonous—though not in the virtually nonexistent quantity that remedies contain.

THE BOTTOM LINE: The notions that you cure a problem by taking what causes it, or that diluting a substance makes it more powerful, are completely at odds with established medical and scientific thinking. As a result, many doctors (and others) say homeopathy doesn't make sense—or can't be explained. Still, a number of studies have raised questions. One controversial study in the respected journal *Nature* documented a white blood cell reacting to a homeopathic dilution of an antibody. A more recent paper in *The Lancet*, a British medical journal, found homeopathy to be more effective than a placebo in three studies of hay fever and asthma. Homeopathy is far from proved, however, and the medical community remains highly skeptical.

AROMATHERAPY: THE NOSE KNOWS

Most people know that smells can have powerful emotional effects. For example, the Monell Chemical Senses Center in Philadelphia recently documented how the distinctive, lingering smell in lower Manhattan after the World Trade Center attacks can trigger depression in residents familiar with it. Smell has pos-

CAUTION

In some cases, homeopathic treatments seem to make symptoms briefly worse before they get better. Homeopaths see this as good because it indicates they've chosen the right remedy, but check with a doctor if you experience unexplained symptoms or suffer more pain. If you use homeopathy, avoid essential oils (used in aromatherapy and massage), which are thought to interact with homeopathic remedies.

itive effects as well—think of the perfumed letter from a lover, or the scent of wildflowers in springtime.

Aromatherapy goes one better, using essential oils distilled or extracted from aromatic plants to treat physical as well as emotional conditions, including various forms of pain. The oils are either inhaled through the nose (often with the help of a diffuser or atomizer that disperses the oil into the air) or rubbed in diluted form onto the skin during a massage. They can also be added to bath water or used in a compress. The theory is that inhaled oils stimulate parts of the brain that govern the body's hormones, while massaged oils enter the bloodstream through the skin. Both routes purportedly influence emotional, mental, and physical health.

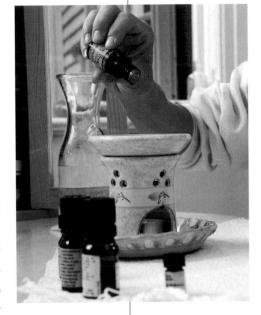

THE BOTTOM LINE: Research supports the idea that aromas can affect emotions, though people often have different reactions to a given smell. Some studies suggest aromatherapy can make you feel calmer and more relaxed, but these effects could easily come from the massage that's often part of the therapy. While undoubtedly pleasant, aromatherapy isn't entirely benign: Essential oils, often made from herbs, can come in extremely potent concentrations. Don't take them internally, and only apply them to the skin following package directions.

MAGNET THERAPY: THE POSITIVES AND NEGATIVES

You don't notice it, but you're awash in magnetic fields: They blanket the earth and help hold the very atoms of your body together. Tiny amounts of magnetic energy lend power to a wide range of processes in the body, including cell division and energy exchange, the pumping of the heart, and transmission of signals through the nervous system.

Even before all this was understood, people used magnets to treat pain and illness—an idea that lost favor in the U.S. in the early 20th century but has recently revived. Adherents say wearing magnets on your body, putting magnetic inserts in your shoes, or using magnetic pillows, mattresses, or car-seat covers influences the body's magnetic fields to promote healing and ease pain. However, it's unclear exactly how magnets might

CAUTION

Magnets are generally assumed to be safe, but their effects on the body aren't well understood, so it's prudent to take reasonable precautions. Don't use magnets if you have a pacemaker or insulin pump, or if you're pregnant. Some experts also advise against using strong magnets on the head, around cancer sites, or on infections.

help. Perhaps they affect the movement of ions (electrically charged particles) as they move in and out of cells. Or maybe magnets boost the body's production of painkilling endorphins. Or, skeptics say, perhaps they do nothing at all.

THE BOTTOM LINE: Magnet therapy isn't well studied, but what little research exists is mixed. A double-blinded, placebo-controlled study in 1999, for example, found that wearing magnetic insoles helped ease burning foot pain for people with diabetes. Of five other well-designed studies, three have found magnets helpful for various types of pain—but two have not.

Supplement Soup

Dietary supplements containing herbs, nutrients, and other substances have soared in popularity, and shelves at health-food stores are loaded with pills and elixirs that claim to relieve pain or conditions that cause it. Do they work? Unfortunately, because supplements are unregulated, they're not required to meet any federal standards for effectiveness or safety. That leaves the responsibility for sorting claims and evidence to consumers.

Experts who look at supplements objectively say products need to be evaluated case-by-case: Some products may be effective at relieving pain or fighting underlying conditions, while others are worthless. The fact that some supplements indeed have clear effects is also reason for caution: It's not unusual for supplements to interact dangerously with other medications or cause side effects of their own. Check with your doctor before taking a supplement, especially if you plan to use it on a regular basis.

WISE BUYS

The supplement industry essentially works on the honor system: Products are unregulated, so you have to trust manufacturers to actually provide what packages promise they contain. But even among honorable makers, quality can vary. To help ensure you're getting the best products:

■ Buy from bigger companies with national distribution: Studies suggest they're generally better at quality control than smaller operations.

■ With multiple brands of a given supplement often available, try to find out what was used in studies showing a benefit, then use the same product yourself.

■ Check labels for clues that a company follows good manufacturing practices. Look for a botanical name if the product is plant-based, a batch or lot number, an expiration date, the manufacturer's address, and information stating the product uses standardized extracts.

OPPOSING OSTEOARTHRITIS

Some of the most popular supplements on the market are promoted (sometimes vaguely, using terms like "joint health," in compliance with rules about health claims) as treatments for osteoarthritis. While the jury is still out on their effectiveness, research to date suggests they may have something to offer.

Glucosamine and Chondroitin: Joint Effort

What if you could take a pill that not only eased the pain of osteoarthritis, but also repaired the damage from the wear and tear that makes joints degenerate? That's the promise of glucosamine sulfate (a simple molecule related to glucose, the main sugar found in blood) and chondroitin sulfate (a natural component of cartilage, the tough connective tissue found in joints). As building blocks of cartilage, the two supplements are either combined or taken individually to treat joint pain.

Though it's too soon to call these supplements a cure for osteoarthritis (as some enthusiasts claim), intriguing evidence suggests they may help. For example, a 2002 study of more than 200 osteoarthritis patients in Britain found glucosamine relieved joint pain as well as ibuprofen—but without the side effects typical with NSAIDs. Other studies observe that such improvements seem to last weeks after patients stop taking glucosamine, suggesting it may go beyond symptom relief to actually repair joints—or at least keep them from deteriorating. Similar claims are made for chondroitin.

So far, these claims are unproven, and not all the research is positive. For example, another 2002 British study found glucosamine no more effective than a placebo at relieving osteoarthritis pain in 80 patients. But many researchers feel these supplements deserve further study in much larger clinical trials.

SAMe: Cartilage Control Plus

Claims like those for glucosamine and chondroitin have also been made for SAMe—short for S-adenosylmethionine. This naturally occurring compound (pronounced "Sammy"), is present in all living cells and affects more than 100 biochemical processes in the body, including cartilage building. SAMe supplements are said to ease joint pain, repair damaged joints, and relieve depression. Because antidepressants are sometimes used to treat fibromyalgia, some people also take SAMe to treat that condition.

SAMe appears to be safe, especially compared with NSAID pain relievers, which some studies suggest SAMe matches in effectiveness. As with glucosamine and chondroitin, it's thought that SAMe somehow affects the osteoarthritis disease process, though the exact mechanism isn't clear. The evidence suggesting SAMe relieves pain is strong enough to win a statement of guarded support from the Arthritis Foundation. Still, SAMe's benefits are unproven, and its high cost—which can hit upward of $200 a month—makes it prohibitively expensive for many people.

Other Contenders

The trio of glucosamine, chondroitin, and SAMe aren't alone in claiming benefits for arthritis. Among the other players are:

Niacinamide. This compound is a basic component of vitamin B_3 (niacin), which the body needs in order to form dozens of enzymes. Niacin is well researched as a treatment for conditions such as high cholesterol, but a 1996 study also found that osteoarthritis patients who took niacinamide showed marked improvement of their symptoms after 12 weeks, while people in a control group got worse. One caution: Subjects in the study took 3,000 mg daily—a high dose that raises a risk of liver inflammation.

JOINT NUTRIENTS

Several substances that help the body build and repair cartilage have become popular supplements for people with joint problems. Preliminary studies in the United States and Europe are encouraging, suggesting that these substances can relieve osteoarthritis symptoms, for example, and may even slow its progress. Side effects appear to be minimal. It often takes several weeks for any of these supplements to produce noticeable benefits, so be patient. On the other hand, if you don't see improvement after two months, assume the supplements are ineffective for you.

Glucosamine

Derived from shrimp, crab, and oyster shells, glucosamine is taken three times a day in doses of 500 mg for pain relief. It is often combined with chondroitin. Diabetics should avoid it.

Chondroitin

This supplement comes from meat gristle, and like glucosamine, should be taken three times a day in doses of 400 or 500 mg. It is often taken with glucosamine.

S-adenosylmethionine (SAMe)

A by-product of a protein the body uses to maintain cartilage, SAMe (pronounced "Sammy") has a typical therapeutic dose of 400 mg three times a day. If you feel the supplement is having an effect, try cutting the dose in half after a few weeks. SAMe also counters mild depression

Caution: Consider avoiding glucosamine if you have diabetes. Animal studies suggest it makes insulin resistance worse.

Phenylalanine. This amino acid occurs naturally in the body, where it contributes to production of key chemicals that transmit signals between nerve cells. In a number of preliminary studies, a synthetic version known as D-phenylalanine has been shown to relieve pain, especially from arthritis. Though it does not affect the basic disease, it may inhibit an enzyme that breaks down the body's natural painkillers. Unfortunately, much of the research on phenylalanine has been scientifically flawed, but results justify further studies.

INHIBITING INFLAMMATION

Reducing inflammation (and thereby easing the pain that goes with it) is the whole point of nonsteroidal anti-inflammatory drugs. But given their nasty side effects and the cost of new medications like COX-2 drugs, are there natural alternatives? Herbalists say yes, though the effects of natural anti-inflammatories are sometimes based more on reputation than solid research. Among the contenders:

Boswellia. Gum resins made from the boswellia tree, which grows in the hills of India, have long been used in traditional Indian herbal medicine to treat both osteoarthritis and rheumatoid arthritis, along with conditions such as bursitis and respiratory diseases. A number of studies, most of them done in India on rheumatoid arthritis, have shown significant reductions of swelling and pain in people taking boswellia—typically in doses of 400 mg, three times daily. These results are highly preliminary, however. Boswellia appears to be safe, though its side effects haven't been comprehensively studied.

Bromelain. In Europe, where herbal remedies are often part of standard medical practice, doctors use this pineapple extract to reduce swelling and inflammation, especially in people recovering from athletic injuries or surgery. They're supported by Germany's Commission E, a scientific review board, which has approved bromelain for sinus inflammation in particular. Still, according to the commission, of five good studies on bromelain, three showed it to be an effective inflammation fighter but two did not, and other scientists have questioned its approval.

Devil's claw. This plant from southern Africa, named for the hooks that cover its fruit, is widely used in Europe to treat joint pain, as well as headache and neuralgia. Studies suggest that compounds in devil's claw have anti-inflammatory properties,

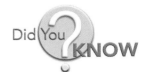

but researchers don't understand how they work. According to Commission E, most studies of devil's claw are poorly designed and have produced mixed results. However, two of the best studies showed supplements produced significant relief for arthritis and low-back pain. Despite its scary name, devil's claw has no known side effects in the typical dose of 750 mg three times a day.

Fish oil. The oils found in fatty, cold-water fish are rich in omega-3 fatty acids, which—though most famous for helping to prevent heart disease—have been shown in studies to reduce inflammation and help ease pain from rheumatoid arthritis. The catch: Benefits are modest, and you have to take large doses (usually 4 to 6 grams per day) over long periods of time (at least six

WEIGHING THE EVIDENCE

Any self-respecting supplement manufacturer will say "studies find" a product works. Whether you can respect these claims is another story. How can you tell if research passes scientific muster?

First, find copies of real studies or abstracts rather than taking the word of marketing material. Start at www.nlm.nih.gov, the National Library of Medicine's website. Apply the same critical standards scientists use:

How big was the study?

Everyone's different, and individuals can vary in their response to treatments. Studies with small numbers of people are vulnerable to the vagaries of variation, while big studies leave less to statistical chance.

Were humans involved?

Animal tests provide important clues and preliminary results that indicate whether studies should be done in real people. But what works in a rat's body may not work in yours.

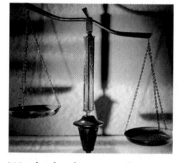

Was it placebo-controlled?

The best studies use two groups of test subjects—one that gets the real treatment and one that gets a fake—so results can be objectively compared. People often get better because they think they will, so good studies make an effort to show treatment produces better results than a placebo.

Was it double-blinded?

Naturally, to control for the placebo effect, subjects shouldn't

know whether they're getting the real treatment or not. Better yet, doctors shouldn't know either. That prevents them from giving it away, perhaps through body language or subtle clues about their expectations.

Was it randomized?

Researchers shouldn't choose which subjects get which treatments, lest they bias the results by picking people they think will skew one way or the other. Instead, subjects should be randomly assigned to groups.

Was it peer-reviewed?

The best studies are published in medical journals that pass muster with editors and with other experts who go over the results with a critical eye on how the study was conducted.

months) to see improvement. Taking that much high-calorie fish oil can make you gain weight, inhibit blood clotting (one of its cardiovascular effects), and cause fishy burps. Possible alternatives to fish oil are fatty acids from plants, such as those in evening primrose oil, but plant oils are not as well studied for pain—and you still have to swallow a lot of oil to gain any benefit.

Stinging nettle. In the wild, stinging nettle lives up to its name: Brushing against the plant's hairy stem or leaves can cause burning pain. As medicine, however, the ancient Greeks used it to treat bites and stings, and Native Americans used it to help with pregnancy and childbirth. Today, nettle is most commonly used to treat prostate enlargement, but popular accounts claim it also works as an anti-inflammatory. There's very little research on whether oral nettle supplements relieve pain. However, researchers at a British medical school in 2002 conducted a controlled, 12-week trial in which they applied nettle leaf topically to aching thumb joints in patients with osteoarthritis.

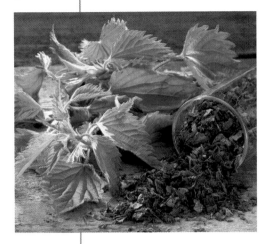

Result: After one week, patients getting nettle treatment had significantly less pain and disability.

Turmeric. You might know it best from your spice rack, but this member of the ginger family has long been used throughout the Eastern world to treat digestive problems such as ulcers, along with a range of other conditions. In the 1970s, researchers in India found evidence that turmeric had anti-inflammatory properties, and natural healers now often recommend it for arthritis as well. (Some products combine it with bromelain.) If it works, turmeric promises anti-inflammatory pain relief that actually heals the stomach rather than irritating it. But so little reliable research has been done on turmeric that these benefits are still largely hearsay.

SEDATIVES AND MOOD MANAGERS

A number of supplements promise to help manage pain by providing psychological rather than physical relief—easing the symptoms of depression and anxiety that often cast a pall over people with chronic pain. Among them:

St. John's wort. One of the best known and most popular herbal remedies, St. John's wort (named for the plant's yellow flower, which blooms around the feast day of St. John) was once

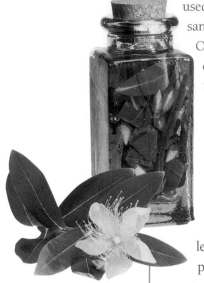

used to cast out demons. Today it's a prescription antidepressant in Germany, with an unusually solid scientific record. One 2002 review of all pertinent studies in the past decade concluded that taking St. John's wort wards off mild to moderate depression just as well as drugs such as Prozac—in some studies, even better. At the same time, St. John's wort has fewer side effects than antidepressant medications. That doesn't make it benign, however: Short-term side effects may include dry mouth, dizziness, sensitivity to sunlight, and gastrointestinal distress—and long-term side effects are not well studied. The FDA warns that St. John's wort can make a wide range of other medications less effective. Typical doses range from 300 mg to 1,000 mg per day, but check with your doctor before taking St. John's wort, especially if you're also taking other drugs for depression.

Kava. In the South Seas, kava has been a social drink for centuries, renowned for its relaxing properties. In the 1960s scientists discovered it contained compounds called kavalactones that have sedative properties, and now it's often used to treat anxiety. One 2002 review of studies from around the world, screened for scientific quality, found seven acceptable studies that found kava better than a placebo at relieving mental stress.

As with St. John's wort, effectiveness means it warrants caution. Though it's generally considered safer than anti-anxiety drugs, you shouldn't mix kava with other drugs, including over-the-counter antihistamines, that are also sedating. Children and pregnant or nursing women should avoid kava, and you should not use it when driving. In 2002 the FDA warned of case reports in which kava appeared to cause liver damage, and the American Herbal Products Association now recommends checking with a doctor before using kava if you've ever had liver problems, frequently drink alcohol, or take any medication.

Valerian. This herb has been used since ancient Greek times to help people sleep—still its main use today. Some studies suggest it works by controlling the brain's use of gamma-aminobutyric acid (GABA), an amino acid that appears related to anxiety, so it's also sometimes taken as a sedative. Valerian is famous for its foul odor, however, so many people prefer kava, whose effectiveness against anxiety has been better demonstrated in studies. Valerian appears to be safe, though the same precautions about sedatives that hold for kava apply to valerian as well.

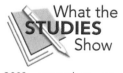

What the
STUDIES
Show

In 2002 researchers at the University of Surrey, in England, tested the effect of valerian and kava on mental stress. Subjects took a stressful-task test, then broke into three groups: one taking kava, one taking valerian, and a control group. A week later they took another test. Results: Those taking kava and valerian performed just as well on the second test as on the first but reported less pressure than the control group.

128

Changing Methods, Changing Minds

It came on gradually—a nagging pain in the hip that started flaring up around the time Nicole Smith* gave birth to twins when she was 35. A physical fitness instructor who taught aerobics and kickboxing in the Boston area, Smith didn't let the discomfort slow her down—at first. But as time went by, the pain continued getting worse, and Smith, now 40, began a long journey seeking relief through a variety of doctors, physical therapists, orthopedists, and chiropractors. "It took a long time," she says, "just to get a proper diagnosis," which was that the pain was originating in a joint connecting her spine to her pelvis.

She eventually settled in with a well-known sports medicine doctor, who prescribed a variety of treatments ranging from physical therapy to wearing a back brace for three months—even acupuncture. "He was great, but after two years, I still didn't have significant relief," Smith says. "I had trouble sitting for more than 20 minutes at a time and wasn't able to sleep through the night." At that point, the doctor referred Smith to Spaulding Rehabilitation Hospital in Boston, where pain treatment includes a variety of alternative therapies.

At Spaulding, she immediately started a multidisciplinary regimen that included gentle manipulation by an osteopath—and acupuncture. "I told my doctor at Spaulding that I'd tried acupuncture before and it didn't do anything," Smith says. "But he said they'd be using a Japanese rather than a Chinese technique." During her treatment, she says, her practitioner (who was also her doctor) asked her many questions, most often trying to determine whether pressing on certain points in her abdomen affected her pain. "The idea was to find acupoints suited to the individual rather than using the same points that are used on everyone else," Smith says. She was still skeptical. "I didn't believe it would help."

Three to four weeks later, however, she'd had a change of heart. "The pain feels much better," she says. "There wasn't an instant difference. I just became aware that I wasn't noticing the nagging pain so much, and I can function much better." Now she can sit comfortably through dinner or a movie and, with the help of a low-dose antidepressant, sleeps through the night. Meanwhile, her osteopathic treatment and physical therapies such as stretching and yoga are working to correct what appear to be structural problems in her hip that are contributing to her pain. "It's hard to know which therapy is helping most," she says. "All the treatments seem to be working together with each other."

* Name has been changed to protect privacy.

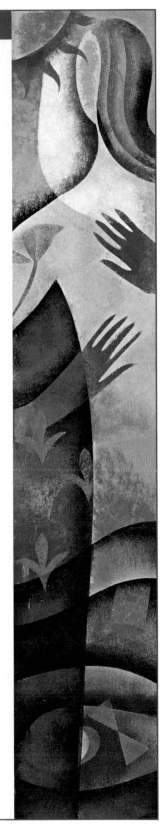

6

COPING
WITH PAIN

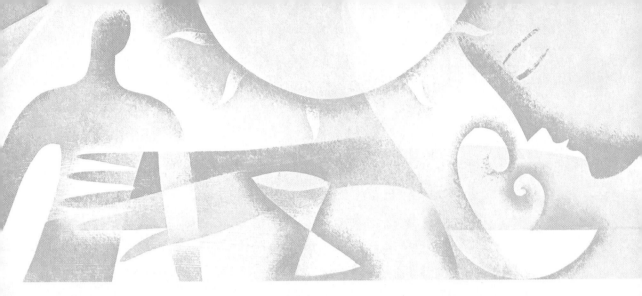

Chronic pain—because it lasts so long and hurts so much—can be understandibly debilitating, causing sufferers to take to their beds and fall into a not unreasonable depression. Pain management doctors are learning that this needn't be the end result of chronic pain. They now encourage patients to try many avenues for relief — from drugs to biofeedback, physical fitness to cognative therapy—to get back to the activities and social relationships that they used to enjoyed.

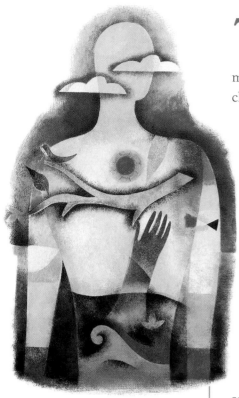

Thomas Jefferson once wrote in a letter that "the art of life is the art of avoiding pain." But when pain becomes unavoidable, what happens to the art of life? Jefferson may not have addressed the point, but millions of people in chronic pain deal with this question day after day.

Doctors are starting to deal with the question as well. Once attuned mainly to medical outcomes, pain specialists (and other physicians) increasingly recognize that the well-being of people with chronic conditions hinges on far more than physical problems or discomfort.

Take the case of arthritis sufferers. In a recent survey of more than 32,000 adults, those with arthritis reported being in poor-to-fair health three times more often than other people did. Maybe that's not surprising when you're talking about the top cause of disability in the United States. But the survey went beyond how arthritis affected people physically to ask how they felt mentally and how often their condition prevented them from participating in regular activities—in short, how well they were coping and getting along. In both cases, people who had arthritis again suffered more than people who didn't.

Such findings point to the importance of what's come to be called health-related quality of life. It's a concept that considers not only the medical measures of your condition—whether you give your pain a 3 or a 7, for example, or how far you can bend your knee—but emotional, social, and other subjective aspects of life as well. It may seem abundantly self-evident that quality of life erodes when you're in constant discomfort. But in many cases, pain chips away so slowly at function, feelings, and favorite activities that patients aren't aware of how—or how much—life has changed. For example, if you've given up tennis because of knee pain, it may not strike you that other enjoyable activities that once seemed important, such as attending matches as a spectator, have also fallen by the wayside.

"Nobody suffering from chronic pain is going to be happy and satisfied about that," says Michael R. Clark, M.D., director of the chronic pain treatment program at Johns Hopkins University School of Medicine's department of psychiatry and behavioral medicine. "The question is what you want out of life and what you can change to make your quality of life better."

Breaking Emotional Barriers

Quality of life isn't strictly about pain itself. Instead, it's about how you react to your pain. You can expect pain to take an emotional toll: That's normal, maybe even inevitable. But people respond to pain differently, and research makes clear that some ways of responding lead to less pain and better outcomes than others.

To get an idea of how you're responding to pain, Clark suggests you think about the goals you may have established for your life. "For people who aren't in pain, this is relatively easy," he says. "They're usually established in careers and relationships, and it's second nature when they wake up in the morning to know what they're striving for and where they're heading. People with chronic pain, on the other hand, often feel that life is passing them by. Their only goal is to get through the day. Often they wonder, 'Is this all life can be?'"

The answer, according to Clark: There's more. "You have opportunities for success and fulfillment, but if you're in chronic pain, you may need to think more assertively about what you need to achieve your goals." These goals may be different now than they were before pain saddled you. But evaluating how to reach them is no different: Look objectively at your strengths and weaknesses (perhaps including personality, skills, and education), and try to identify activities or ambitions that match your capabilities. Sound like a familiar process? Then the next question becomes critical: What's holding you back?

For many people in chronic pain, the answer comes down to emotional barriers. These may include depression, anxiety, anger, or loss of self-esteem, along with issues these negative feelings become entangled with, such as weight gain and deteriorating relationships—all of which can make pain more difficult to deal with and quality of life more difficult to achieve.

THE PATHOS OF PAIN

If pain takes some emotional stuffing out of you, you've got good reason to feel the way you do—and plenty of company. A variety of studies have documented how pain often makes it more difficult to perform (or keep) a job, grinds your social gears, and

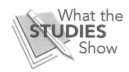

may rob you of your regular roles at work, at home, and in the community. "In certain ways, it's like grief," says Clark. "You're dealing with loss—of health, of function, of identity." As such, you can expect to go through several distinct stages, similar to those made famous by psychiatrist Elisabeth Kübler-Ross, the noted authority on grief and death:

■ **Denial.** You find it hard to believe how things have changed, and may feel a bit numb.

■ **Anger.** Disbelief turns to bitterness as you grapple with the reality of your pain, perhaps wondering what you did to "deserve" it, or seeking sources of blame for your discomfort.

■ **Depression.** You feel sad about your condition and the prospect of continuing to deal with it.

■ **Acceptance.** While pain never exactly becomes "acceptable," you nevertheless learn to live with it and make the most of your life despite whatever limitations you may have.

Not everyone goes through all these stages—or experiences them in the same order, says Clark. The important thing is that you continue moving toward acceptance without getting mired at any one point. Emotions like depression, anger, and anxiety are common in people with chronic pain, but lingering psychological distress shouldn't be complacently accepted as normal and inevitable—just as physical pain shouldn't be dismissed as a normal element of chronic illness. "The key is how well you're functioning," says Clark. "If psychological suffering becomes debilitating, you deserve treatment for it at least as much as someone who doesn't also have chronic pain."

HOW TO PROBLEM-SOLVE PAIN

It's easy to think the worst when pain flares up, but doctors find "catastrophizing" to be one of the least helpful ways to cope with suffering. For starters, thoughts like "It's terrible and I feel it's never going to get better" won't provide you with any relief. But beyond that, studies find negative thinking, excessive worrying, and focusing on fear actually lead to poorer outcomes over time than dealing with pain in a more positive way.

How can you be positive about pain? Doctors find that people tend to do better when they deal with pain as a series of distinct issues rather than as a single overwhelming problem. Breaking your difficulties into smaller pieces makes it easier to

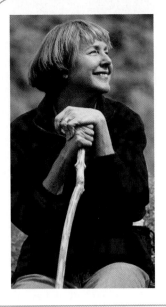

CHANGING YOUR MIND

A growing number of studies find that what you believe, expect, and think about pain can help or hinder your efforts to cope, depending on what goes through your mind.

To make useful changes in your point of view, pain specialists say you're best off developing a take-charge approach that builds on these key ideas:

▷ You're not a passive victim when it comes to pain. You may listen to your pain, but you have something to say as well—and you're the one in charge.

▷ Though it's natural for your physical condition, moods, and various environmental factors to affect your thinking, strong positive beliefs can help you physically, mentally, and socially.

▷ It's possible to learn better ways of thinking, feeling, and behaving so that pain seems manageable, not overwhelming.

come up with practical solutions that seem more manageable. To take a problem-solving approach:

▶ **Consider the impact** pain has on different areas of your life, such as job, family, social situations, recreation, finances, and physical condition. Think of each area as a separate set of problems, and list the specific challenges you face one by one.

▶ **Fine-tune your understanding** of what leads to challenges in each area. Think in descriptive terms such as, "When this happens in that situation, I feel this way." Work to identify specific scenarios that you associate with pain, perhaps with the help of a pain diary.

▶ **Try to think how you might change** various scenarios to get a better outcome. Could you take your medication at a different time or in a different dose? Have you been pushing yourself too hard? Can you pace your activities better? Are there certain people you'd be better off avoiding? Are there other therapies you might try?

▶ **Think in action terms** using words like "catch," "interrupt," "choices," and "experiment." Then come up with a plan.

▶ **Put your ideas into action.** Understand from the start that no single solution is likely to solve any given problem, so you'll need to try different ideas. If one approach doesn't work, don't see it as a failure, but as a learning experience that will help you in the future.

Dealing with Depression

The "D" word comes up repeatedly when talking about emotions and pain, with good reason—two, in fact. First, people suffering from chronic discomfort such as low-back pain languish under lingering clouds of gloom (as opposed to normal blues that come and go) three to four times as much as the general population. But just as important, depression appears to intensify pain.

In rheumatoid arthritis patients, for example, studies have linked depression with severity of pain over the course of many days, even when the arthritis itself doesn't get worse and people aren't any more disabled. Depression and pain are so closely entwined, they create a chicken-and-egg dilemma: Does pain cause depression or does depression cause pain? Researchers are still working out the connection, but emphasize that, while they're related, pain and depression are separate beasts—and you can treat or manage them both.

Everybody has occasional bouts with the blues, but there's a difference between a run-of-the-mill slump and being gripped by dark feelings that cling like shackles. When low moods don't go away, that's not just a state of mind, it's a clinical condition.

CHASING THE BLUES AWAY

Though depression is often triggered by events in life, being in pain may not be the only reason you feel down. "People often passively assume that if the pain goes away, the depression will too," says Clark. "But that's not necessarily the case." In fact, a variety of factors can contribute to depression, including genetics, chemical imbalances in the brain, and hormonal disruptions. Fortunately, you can treat depression in a variety of ways.

Antidepressant Medications

Antidepressants are the front-line defense against the blues, especially with chronic pain, because they lift moods and, in many cases, do double duty as potent analgesics. Four major classes of medications are:

Tricyclics. Drugs such as Elavil, Pamelor, Norpramin, and Tofranil lift mood by boosting levels of natural chemicals found in the brain and spinal cord such as serotonin and norepinephrine. Before newer medications such as Prozac hit the market around the early 1990s, tricyclic antidepressants were the blues-battling treatment of choice. Today (as noted in chapter 2), they're just as likely to be tapped first for pain relief, which kicks in faster and at lower doses than any mood-lifting effects. Some people taking these drugs experience side effects such as dry mouth, weight gain, sedation, and low blood pressure.

Atypical drugs. Drugs like Effexor, Serzone, Wellbutrin, Remeron, and the newest, duloxetine, bridge the gap between the tricyclics and the SSRIs, working in much the same way and offering some evidence of pain relief.

SSRIs. Best known by brand names such as Prozac, Paxil, and Zoloft, selective serotonin reuptake inhibitors help to maintain adequate levels of serotonin in the brain. These newest antidepressants are likely to be the first choice for treating depression, partly because they tend to have milder side effects than older drugs. However, they don't appear to relieve pain as well as tricyclics, and side effects such as nervousness, insomnia, lack of appetite, and lower sex drive still affect some people.

MAO inhibitors. Monoamine oxidase inhibitors such as Nardil and Parnate block the action of an enzyme that breaks down mood-improving chemicals such as norepinephrine and dopamine. Though they've also been found to have pain-relieving properties, they can cause serious side effects such as high blood pressure and heart rate, and difficulty breathing. As a result, they're usually prescribed only when other antidepressants don't work.

Psychotherapy

Don't let the word put you off: You don't have to have a mental illness to benefit from psychotherapy, or talk-based treatments in which a trained mental health professional helps you

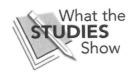

What the STUDIES Show

One hallmark of catastrophizing is fearing your pain will only get worse. But deterioration isn't inevitable. One study that followed up on chronic pain patients from family practices and pain clinics for two years found at the end of that period:

> A substantial number of patients had no pain at all.

> Those who continued to experience pain found it became more intermittent.

> Emotional distress over pain diminished dramatically.

> Patients needed substantially fewer medical services.

CAN PAIN BE A PLUS?

Some people who cope well with pain are blessed with strong personal or social resources—say, a naturally sunny disposition or a caring family. But sometimes, people with none of those blessings also take a dispassionate view of pain that makes it easier to deal with. One way to explain the overlap: Paradoxically, doctors find that pain sometimes provides a focus for people whose lives are stressful, chaotic, or unsatisfactory. In some cases, pain allows patients to ignore other challenges, providing what might strangely be described as a form of relief from problems they may see as worse.

READING THE SIGNS

How can you tell the difference between a passing thunderstorm and a never-ending drizzle when it all looks like rain? It's somewhat more difficult to diagnose clinical depression in people with chronic pain because the two conditions sometimes share physical symptoms. But according to diagnostic criteria from the American Psychiatric Association, you may have depression if five or more of the following are true for at least two straight weeks:

✪ You feel sad, anxious, or irritable almost all of the time.

✪ You don't take much interest or pleasure in many—if any—daily activities.

✪ You feel worthless or guilty.

✪ You have more—or less—of an appetite than usual, or you've gained—or lost—a significant amount of weight.

✪ You lack energy.

✪ You feel agitated or sluggish in your responses.

✪ You find it difficult to concentrate or make decisions.

✪ You have trouble sleeping—or you sleep more than usual.

✪ You often find yourself thinking about death or suicide.

understand—and feel better about—your thoughts, emotions, and behavior.

One major form of psychotherapy is interpersonal therapy, which tries to overcome depression by helping you understand and improve your relationships. Among the issues a therapist might explore with you (typically in 12 to 15 sessions) are conflicts with other people, unresolved grief, difficulties moving from one position in life to another, and development of people skills.

A second form of psychotherapy is cognitive-behavioral therapy, in which you learn to recognize and replace negative, irrational thoughts with positive, rational ones. It's a perception/reality game. For example:

Perception: Something bad happened. It must be my fault.
Reality: It probably has nothing to do with you.

Perception: I can't do everything I used to. I'm worthless.
Reality: There's a lot you still can do. You can find value in your current abilities.

Perception: I'm unhappy and I can't help it.
Reality: You can take charge of your moods and enjoy life despite your pain.

Perception: Things will never change.
Reality: Nothing stays the same, and your situation could very well improve.

Helping Yourself

Don't let gloomy statistics on pain and depression get you down: Having pain doesn't automatically make you bound for the blues. The fact is, though depression is far more common in people with pain than without, most people experiencing chronic pain are not battling the black dogs of despair.

One large-scale survey of Americans found that only 18 percent of people with chronic pain met the psychiatric criteria for depression, versus 8 percent of the general population—so only a fraction of people with chronic pain experience mental suffering as well.

If, however, you are among the chronic pain sufferers who also must fight depression, there are healing practices you can adopt for yourself. For example, once you have learned psychological techniques like those of cognitive-behavioral therapy (facing page), you can practice them on your own. And they're not the only steps you can take to lift your mood without professional help. Some easy, effective mood-brighteners include:

- **Stepping out.** Rubbing elbows with others in social settings can take your mind off pain, help you gain perspective on your problems, and make you feel less isolated. You don't have to throw a party to make it happen: Simply participating in activities at a social club or religious congregation puts you in the company of like-minded people.
- **Moving your body.** Physical activity is a potent mood-booster that in some studies rivals antidepressant medications. One theory is that exercise raises levels of natural chemicals in the brain that foster feelings of satisfaction and well-being. But physical activity also helps you sleep better, boosts energy, makes you feel more in control of life, and provides a cheering sense of accomplishment.

Alleviating Anger

If being in pain makes you angry, join the crowd. Given incessant discomfort, less-than-perfect treatment, loss of sleep, and lack of understanding from loved ones, co-workers, or insurance companies, it's no wonder frustration is the single most powerful negative emotion people in chronic pain typically feel. If your teeth-gnashing is also marred by depression, you're even more likely to simmer and seethe.

Some researchers suggest that anger in people with chronic pain is underrecognized because patients often deny their feelings.

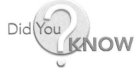

Did You **KNOW**

Why do some people with chronic pain get depressed while many others don't? Depression may be a swirl of psychological, family, and genetic factors, but some cases can at least partially be explained in a more straightforward way. Studies find that depression often directly reflects how much pain interferes with normal activities that are important to people, which limits uplifting social contact and makes sufferers feel less in control of their lives.

Why does this matter? Because hostility hurts your relationships, raises your risk of health problems such as heart disease, and actually intensifies your pain. Don't buy the theory that unbridled venting clears the air and makes you feel better: Studies find that acting out anger actually increases your hostility and makes you more likely to fly off the handle in the future. Some ways to recognize and pacify your passions:

▶ **Tame your triggers.** Chances are, you tend to become annoyed, irritated, or enraged in certain situations over and over. Think of when your anger tends to flare. It could be when you're around specific people, when certain topics come up in conversation, when you're behind the wheel or standing in a checkout line. Knowing in advance what fans your flames can help you avoid situations you know will provoke you and prompt you to think about why you find these scenarios so aggravating. In many cases, simply understanding anger better helps take the edge off.

▶ **Take a step back.** The old advice about counting to 10 makes sense because even a brief irritation interlude gives you a chance to analyze your anger. Why are you upset? Are your grievances legitimate and justified? Is the issue important—really? Is your reaction appropriate? Are you assuming that other people are insulting you or trying to take advantage of you? If you put yourself in the other person's shoes, would the situation look the same way? Challenging your assessments can help you see aggravating situations in a more understanding, less hostile light.

▶ **Win by "losing."** Minor brushfire arguments can quickly escalate into conflagrations simply because nobody backs down. Experts say you can just as quickly dump water on a conflict by doing the unexpected: agreeing with something the other person says. You don't have to concede your entire argument. Just pick one point you can concede to be true. If the other person says, "Your mother drives me crazy," say, "She has her moments, doesn't she?" Your positive (or at least neutral) response sets a positive tone for the rest of the conversation.

▶ **Be direct.** Some anger may be worth expressing if doing so can make a positive difference and the issue is important enough. But that doesn't mean you should go in with both barrels blasting. If, for example, someone has offended you or is doing something you don't like, start by making a simple, specific, matter-of-fact assertion that focuses on you rather than the other person. For example, if someone persistently interrupts you, don't say, "You keep butting in," say, "Excuse me, I'd like to finish what I'm saying."

Resting Easier

When you're pummeled with pain, it's likely your sleep quality is slipping, both because discomfort makes it hard for your body to rest comfortably, and because anxiety keeps your mind firing when it should be calming down. But reclaiming a little slumber can have big benefits. Getting enough rest not only ensures you have adequate energy to meet each day's challenges, it takes the edge off irritability and strengthens your fortitude.

"If you have a good night's sleep, it's easier to cope with just about anything," says Perry Fine, M.D., professor of anesthesiology at the University of Utah Pain Management Center. "But if you have a lousy night's sleep, even trivial things can seem difficult to deal with." In one recent survey that asked patients the ways pain affected daily living, interference with sleep topped the list. "Normalizing sleep patterns is one of the most important steps you can take to enhance quality of life," Fine says.

Often the first step is to get appropriate pain medication to keep physical suffering to a minimum so that you can rest. In some cases, doctors prescribe antidepressants that also cause drowsiness. But regardless of whether you take medications, you will get better-quality shuteye by taking steps like the following:

▶ **Get on a schedule.** Sleep is set by your body clock, but the machinery isn't on full autopilot: You help set the clock through your daily habits. As much as possible, try to schedule regular activities, such as eating meals, at the same times each day, which helps cue your body to the passing of the hours. Most important, go to bed and get up at the same times each day, which tells the body how to regulate sleep-governing processes such as the release of hormones.

▶ **Wind down.** Make a ritual of preparing for bed, which both cues the body that it's time for sleep and calms you down. Relaxing elements of a bedtime ritual might include taking a warm bath, eating a light snack, listening to restful music, or reading a good book.

▶ **Lock out sleep robbers.** You know not to drink coffee just before bed, but try laying off the java by midafternoon: Some research suggests that caffeine still has stimulating effects as long as eight hours later. Beware sneaky sources of caffeine such as chocolate, soft drinks (including some brands of orange soda and root beer), and decaf coffee (which contains small amounts of caffeine). And nix the nightcap: Alcohol

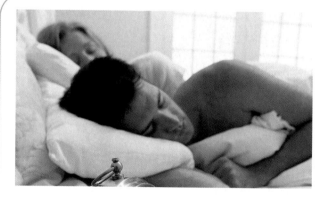

THE AMBIANCE OF DREAMLAND

Experts call it "sleep hygiene," but it has nothing to do with keeping clean. Rather, good sleep often depends on controlling external factors that can interfere with quality slumber. Some easy steps you can take to make your environment more conducive to crashing:

Don't make your bedroom your den. Leave the TV and paperwork elsewhere in the house and reserve the bedroom strictly for sleep and sex.

Negate nocturnal noise. You might get used to soft household noises like the furnace kicking in, but studies suggest that louder, sporadic sounds like passing cars or aircraft probably disrupt sleep more than you sus-

pect. To mask noise, buy a white noise machine or a noise generator that sounds like waves or a babbling brook.

Turn down the thermostat. Cooler temperatures generally induce better sleep.

Dim the lights. Even if you're sleepy, too much light in the room can make dozing difficult. Turn off nightlights, shut the bed-

room door, and put room-darkening shades on the windows.

Don't overlook the obvious. People have different preferences for mattresses and pillows, but the important thing is that yours be comfortable.

Keep the bedroom neat. It'll promote a sense of order and control that can help put your mind at ease.

may help make you nod off, but as it's metabolized in the body, it will disrupt sleep later in the night.

- **Calm your mind.** You can blame most insomnia on having an overactive mind. Often it's due to fretting about your future, your finances, your family, or any number of familiar worries. But paradoxically, you may also be losing sleep worrying about … losing sleep. To keep conscious thoughts from careening into the anxiety zone, try listing your worries before you go to bed, and brainstorm possible solutions. If anxious thoughts intrude while you're trying to drift off, you can tell yourself you've already dealt with those problems. If sleep itself is your concern, don't languish in a fuzzy-headed dusk between sleep and wakefulness for more than 15 minutes. Instead, get up and do something calm and quiet, like reading something dull. Go to bed only when you feel drowsy again.

- **Spend less time in bed.** If you're chronically short on shut-eye, you'd think spending more moments under the covers would get you back on track. But too much time in bed may actually make your sleep more shallow and less restful. Instead, try going to bed later (when you're actually tired) and rising earlier. You may get fewer hours of sleep, but you'll probably snooze more soundly.

Rebuilding Relationships

For some people, chronic pain can seem to make a train wreck of life—a slow-motion pileup of frustration, anger, and depression. But even without the negative emotions, pain can strain relationships with people around you, particularly the family members and friends with whom you're closest. Few social bonds make it through this crucible without fraying at least a little, but it's possible to keep relationships on track by bearing some simple principles in mind.

First, it's natural for those who care about you most to want to help. No problem there. But try to be patient with people if you find what they do to be less helpful than they imagine. Be open about your real needs, and offer matter-of-fact suggestions about what you find most beneficial. Encourage loved ones to learn more about your pain so they can understand better what you're going through. You can play a role in helping to educate them: When they ask how you're doing, don't gloss over your pain, but don't exaggerate it either. Explain what you feel, how it changes, and how you're learning to deal with it.

Most of all, try to live a normal life in which you do as much for yourself as possible. Ask people for help when you need it, but don't let them (or yourself) dwell on your pain, which may just make you feel worse. Expect there to be some friction (especially if you're spending more time with loved ones), but recognize that having social support is linked to better pain management. Here's how to keep the social gears well oiled:

THE GOOD FIGHT

Most people try to avoid conflicts, but you shouldn't necessarily squelch squabbles with friends or—especially—significant others: Happy couples actually fight more, not less, than unhappy ones. The difference is that people in healthy relationships resolve more problems. Some finer points of fighting well:

Don't jump to solutions. The real issue and the thing you're fighting about often aren't the same. It's a mistake to problem-solve too quickly when one or both parties simply want their feelings heard. Let sometimes trivial arguments unravel for a while to let deeper issues such as rejection and fear percolate to the surface.

Back off, but don't go. It's healthy to take a step back for a time-out if passions are burning too hot and the fight is going nowhere. But it doesn't help to storm out the door and leave the argument hanging before it's been resolved. If you're tak-

ing off, tell your partner when the conversation will resume—and follow up.

Look for common ground. Differences can obscure shared values. Work to discover where you agree, then start building bridges.

Take feelings seriously. They might not make sense. They could strike you as irrational. But even if you don't understand, you need to value and respect the other person's emotions.

Keep the past in the past. You won't get any closer to resolving an argument today by dredging

up conflicts from last week. If you still need to address unresolved issues, save them for another time.

Problem-solve as a pair. Together, try to find as many solutions to the real problem as possible. Decide to pursue the best ideas and work out the concrete steps you'll take to do it.

Sign a truce. Communicate to each other that you've reached a resolution—or at least have taken things as far as you can for now—and the conflict isn't a barrier between you. The signal could be as simple as a kind word, a hug, or a squeeze of the hand.

- **Gravitate to good.** It's natural to snipe about what irritates you, but everyone around you will feel better if you focus on what's good about a relationship. One way to do it is to practice what some therapists call the three A's:

  - ▸ **Appreciation.** Tell loved ones the qualities you like about them, or let them know when they do something that makes you happy. A simple word of thanks, a comment on their thoughtfulness, or a positive observation about their personality—all are expressions of appreciation.

    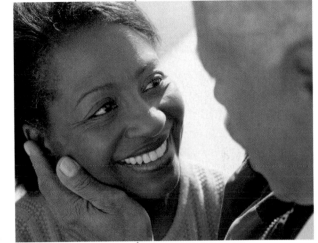

  - ▸ **Affection.** Show signs that you like the people around you—by, for example, touching or hugging, or simply stating your feelings.

  - ▸ **Affirmation.** Let others know that you value them and your relationship, perhaps by making simple statements such as "I'm glad you're my friend" or "I can't imagine getting along without you."

- **Complain constructively.** It can't all be upbeat and affirming: Inevitably, you'll face issues that make you unhappy. To deal with them best, start by crafting your complaints. Never start by launching into a litany of offenses. Instead, focus on one gripe at a time, and be specific. Don't say, "The house is always a mess," say, "I'd feel better if the dishes were washed and put away." Ask for reasonable changes, but be ready to hear the other person's point of view and come up with a compromise.

- **Spend time together.** When you're in pain, it's easy to get wrapped up in the humorless hassles of life. Nevertheless, it's important to do things you enjoy with people you love. This not only shows them you like being with them but gives you an opportunity to deepen your relationship through conversation and distract yourself from your pain.

- **Don't wait to be asked.** If pain hinders your activities, you may find that your social bonds are becoming weaker. Don't make the mistake of assuming that people hate being around you: If friends and acquaintances don't know how much you are (or are not) suffering, they might assume you would rather not be around them. To show them otherwise—and keep your social circle spinning—accept as many invitations as you can. But don't wait for other people to make the first move. Call friends and suggest going for coffee or a movie, take part in community activities such as fairs, festivals, or charitable fund-raisers, or get involved with local social or political organizations.

Stimulating Self-Esteem

If self-esteem strikes you as the stuff of psychobabble and indulgent self-congratulation, you've got the wrong idea. Self-esteem isn't about blowing yourself kisses to make yourself feel good (whether you deserve to or not). Rather, it's about feeling you have the inner strength and competence to meet life's daily challenges. Feeling reined in by pain can chip away at your self-image. But maintaining your inner strength can significantly boost your power to cope with pain.

Central to self-esteem is what psychologists call self-efficacy: the belief that you're capable of doing what's needed to achieve a desired outcome. The higher your self-efficacy, the more likely you are to choose constructive action, put forth effort to meet a goal, persevere in the face of obstacles, fend off depression and anxiety, and move toward accomplishment.

Studies find that people who score high in self-efficacy tend to see demanding situations as challenges and attribute failure to lack of knowledge, skill, or effort—factors that can be developed. People who score low in self-efficacy, on the other hand, see demanding situations as something to avoid, tend to give up more easily, and are more prone to stress and depression. Bottom line, as indicated by studies in osteoarthritis patients, those with high self-efficacy report lower levels of pain and disability than people with low self-efficacy.

Issues of self-esteem and self-efficacy can seem deeply rooted, but they're actually subject to change, especially by working to confront a challenge and meeting with success—what's known as a mastery experience. Some first steps to take on the road to mastery and higher self-esteem:

- **Be critical.** That doesn't mean getting down on yourself. Instead, objectively consider your strengths and weaknesses with the understanding that nobody's perfect. Look, too, at the core beliefs and values that guide your life: Without them, you'll too easily be blown by the winds of self-doubt. Recognize and affirm what you like about yourself. As for the things you don't like, ask yourself what you consider really important to your self-image. Then work to change what you can and ignore what you can't.

- **Take realistic risks.** People with low self-esteem can often be paralyzed by fear of failure. That's not entirely bad: You have to be sensible about what your true limitations are and make prudent choices to ensure success. But success also depends on carefully thinking through alternatives and taking reasonable risks when your chances of succeeding are actually pretty good.

- **See failure as fortunate.** Everybody makes mistakes and suffers setbacks, so don't expect to be any different. The real difference lies in what people do with their failures. The best attitude is to view setbacks as stepping-stones to eventual success: Without them, you won't learn what to do better next time. Each setback and failure that teaches you something makes you stronger, not weaker.

- **Look to tomorrow.** While you can use past setbacks to chart the course ahead, don't dwell on the past—beating yourself up over failures or striving to match past successes. You should always see the starting line as today, and the race lying ahead, not behind.

- **Face rejection.** Self-esteem is partly determined by social signals we get from other people, and it's easy to assume that we must be flawed or worthless when others don't appreciate us. Surprisingly, social scientists say that if you think certain people don't like you, you're probably right. It's simply a fact that people are very different, that various groups have different norms, and that people judge each other by how well they conform to expectations. It's inevitable that someone will find you unacceptable. But their disapproval is their problem, not yours.

◉ **Fudge your feedback.** Recognizing that not everyone's in your camp doesn't mean you have to bunk with those who belittle you. Surround yourself with people who appreciate you and lift you up rather than tear you down. When getting away from people (co-workers, family members) isn't possible, let them know when you feel they're being disrespectful or hurtful. Standing up for yourself is sometimes the first step toward gaining respect.

DECISION-MAKING MADE EASY

Making crisp, clear decisions can be the bane of people who feel low about themselves due to problems with self-esteem or depression. But making up your mind can be easier if you consider the following points:

◉ **It's okay not to rush.** You don't want to procrastinate, but there's nothing wrong with taking your time to consider the pluses and minuses, especially if a decision is likely to have long-term consequences. Go ahead and sleep on it—but be sure to make the decision tomorrow.

◉ **Use a "Does it matter?" meter.** Not every choice is worth losing sleep over. Put the decision in context and don't worry about issues you would objectively judge to be relatively unimportant in the broad scheme of things.

◉ **Don't assume there's one answer.** Fear of making the wrong decision may be holding you back, but most outcomes are mixed, and whatever you decide is likely to be better than not deciding at all.

◉ **Retain the right to re-decide.** Most judgments aren't set in stone. If a decision doesn't work out, you can always make new choices to correct the consequences.

PARING PAINFUL POUNDS

One sometimes overlooked impediment to high quality of life for people in chronic pain is weight gain, which can result from lack of physical activity due to pain, compounded by drags on get-up-and-go such as depression, fatigue, and lack of self-efficacy. It's not a cosmetic issue: Being overweight puts extra stress on muscles and joints, hinders flexibility, and dampens your sense of well-being—all of which may contribute to pain. Putting on pounds also puts you at higher risk for a range of serious conditions such as heart disease and diabetes. Fortunately, it doesn't take dramatic weight loss to significantly improve your risks—losing even a few pounds can make a big difference. Some ways to do it:

- **Police your portions.** You can do this easily at home but eating out these days has become a challenge. Serving sizes in restaurants, have gone from big to gigantic—for example, hamburgers now are commonly twice the size typical 25 years ago. But you're not at the mercy of a restaurant menu: Hors d'oeuvres may be intended as a warm-up, but there's no reason you can't consider them the main course. Another trick is to split a full-portion entrée with a friend.

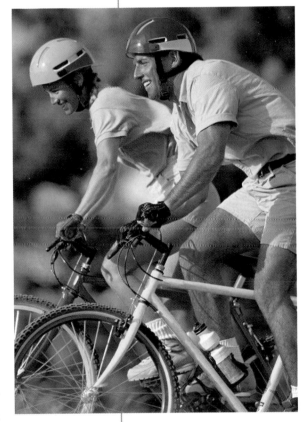

- **Start slow with exercise.** It's important to be physically active, both to condition your body so it more readily resists pain (see chapter 4) and to burn excess calories. However, studies suggest that if you start with overly vigorous aerobic exercise, you may burn calories while you are working out, but tiredness could make you less active than ever for the rest of the day, compromising your gains. Begin your fitness regimen with easy activities like walking, then start gradually exercising more vigorously over the period of a few weeks.

- **Aim for a steady loss**. Don't expect—or try to achieve—dramatic results in a short time: You'll only be disappointed if you don't succeed, and will likely gain back any pounds that you lose quickly. Instead, aim to eat a balanced diet (heavy on grains, fruits, and vegetables and light on red meats and fats) that lets you lose weight gradually—no more than a pound or two a week. Be sure to eat all your meals so hunger doesn't make you overindulge, and allow yourself small amounts of favorite treats—even if they're high in fat.

7

HELP NOW
AND IN THE
FUTURE

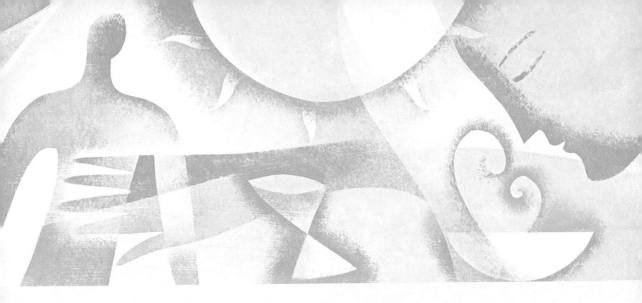

When you have a chronic disease, you must form a partnership with your doctor and, frequently, a whole team of other doctors and technicians. Getting the help you need may take a lot of trial and error; the important point to keep in mind is that everything that doesn't work tells you and your doctors something else about your problem that may ultimately help to solve it. Don't give up the fight; here are some guidelines for making the best use of the new pain management field of medicine.

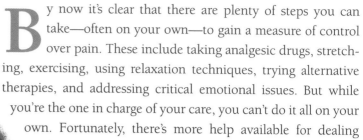

By now it's clear that there are plenty of steps you can take—often on your own—to gain a measure of control over pain. These include taking analgesic drugs, stretching, exercising, using relaxation techniques, trying alternative therapies, and addressing critical emotional issues. But while you're the one in charge of your care, you can't do it all on your own. Fortunately, there's more help available for dealing with pain than ever before.

Most of your help, of course, will—and should—come from doctors, who nevertheless can be a source of both relief and frustration. Chances are, if you're suffering from chronic pain (defined as lasting six months or more), you've already been through your share of general practitioners and specialists. "Patients on average have seen five or six doctors before they get to us," says Vildan Mullin, M.D., director of the Multidisciplinary Pain Center at the University of Michigan Health System, Ann Arbor, which operates one of the nation's largest training programs for pain specialists. "Some patients have seen as many as 15 different doctors."

Organizing Your Team

Pain care is becoming increasingly patient-centered— which means "ownership" of pain falls to you, not your doctor or any therapist. That's best, because only you truly understand your pain, so you need to be the manager of your care. Like any boss, you can't expect to have all the answers yourself. Instead, you need to surround yourself with capable advisers who give you options for the decisions you have to make.

The often intractable nature of pain can be challenging for patients and doctors alike. In one recent survey of more than 1,000 pain patients, 62 percent of those who were unhappy with their doctors cited unsuccessful treatment as the reason they were dissatisfied. There are two lessons in this. First, patients increasingly realize that you shouldn't be content with treatment that doesn't provide relief. Second, and just as important, if your treatment is unsatisfactory, there may be other approaches or other doctors that can help more—especially as the number of doctors and clinics specializing in pain management grows. Continuing to seek relief is the essence of taking charge of your pain: When you can't ease your pain on your own, you marshal a team of experts who can.

With almost a million physicians in the United States, there's no shortage of doctors. The trick is finding those that can help you the most. Given the complexity of pain and the fact that it's a common part of so many different conditions, it helps first to be clear about the different kinds of doctors and how their approach to your care may differ.

THE MEDICAL SQUAD

Not every person in chronic pain will need the same types of people on their pain management team. But players from the medical profession might typically include:

■ **Primary-care physician.** This may be the first doctor you see, often because health insurance plans require that referrals to specialists come through a primary-care doctor. He or she will attempt to diagnose what's causing your pain, and in many cases can prescribe drugs or therapies that will stop it. Primary-care physicians are often generalists, with postgraduate training in fields such as internal medicine, gynecology, pediatrics, and family medicine—but not necessarily in pain or the conditions that cause it. A good primary-care physician will understand the limits of his or her expertise, passing you along to a specialist if a particular condition such as arthritis or cancer warrants it, or if prescribed therapies don't work.

■ **Condition specialist.** Depending on the nature of your pain, you may need the help of a doctor who specializes in the condition causing your pain. Specialists who often deal with chronic pain include:

    ■ **Rheumatologists,** who are trained to diagnose and treat arthritis and other inflammatory or autoimmune conditions affecting the joints and joint tissues.

    ■ **Oncologists,** who specialize in treating cancer, with subspecialties that include medical oncology, radiation oncology, gynecological oncology, and surgical oncology.

    ■ **Orthopedists,** who focus on preserving or restoring the function of the skeletal system, often through surgery.

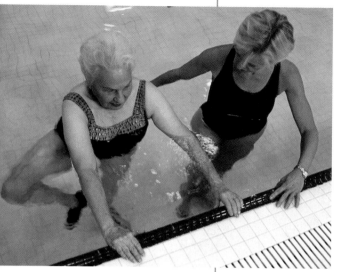

■ **Pain doctor.** Doctors who specialize in painful conditions often see the control of suffering as one of their most important goals for patients. Other doctors who specifically deal with pain, often in specialized clinics, include:

> ■ **Neurologists and neurosurgeons.** They specialize in treating neuropathic pain that arises from the nervous system.
>
> ■ **Anesthesiologists.** These doctors control pain during surgery and also help manage pain more generally, using medications, nerve blocks and other procedures.

■ **Physical therapist.** A PT can prescribe exercises for relieving pain and restoring lost muscle and joint function, using tools such as heat and cold, nerve stimulation, stretching, aerobics, strength exercises, massage, and water therapy.

■ **Occupational therapist.** An OT can help you perform everyday tasks around the home by modifying your surroundings so you can function more effectively, teaching you new ways to get things done, or fitting you with devices that help you perform better.

■ **Mental health specialist.** A psychologist holds a master's or doctoral degree in psychology and is trained to help you deal with stress, manage your emotions, and change negative behavior through counseling, psychotherapy, or cognitive-behavioral therapy. Psychologists can't, however, prescribe medications. Psychiatrists—medical doctors with training in the relationship between mental health and physical well-being—can treat psychological disorders by prescribing medications such as antianxiety drugs or antidepressants.

■ **Support professionals.** Nurses, who may actually be the people you spend the most time with, conduct assessments, monitor your use of medications, and provide you with information. Other professionals you and your doctor might call into service include a social worker to help you cope with family, financial, or work issues; a dietitian to advise you on proper nutrition and weight control; a vocational rehabilitation specialist to focus on return-to-work issues such as job modifications and ergonomics; and perhaps a chaplain, who can help you deal with the spiritual aspects of your condition.

THE COMPLEMENTARY PLAYERS

Should you call in alternative practitioners? That's a call you'll have to make on your own after weighing the evidence supporting the therapies you have in mind, and consulting with your doctor. Though no alternative treatment takes the place of ongoing medical care, many patients might consider including the following professionals in their pain treatment:

■ **Acupuncturist.** Trained in using acupuncture needles to treat pain and other conditions, acupuncturists should meet standards for safety and experience set by the National Certification Commission for Acupuncture and Oriental Medicine or, perhaps even better, be a medical doctor who is

WOMEN AND PAIN

Is pain different for women? It's a hot topic among pain doctors, who—like many in the medical community—are now looking more closely at how gender affects both diseases and their treatments.

For starters, women experience higher rates of painful conditions such as migraines and tension headaches, osteoarthritis and rheumatoid arthritis, fibromyalgia, temporomandibular disorders (TMD), pelvic pain, and abdominal pain. Whether the quality of women's pain differs from that of men is more controversial. Numerous studies suggest that women tend to feel pain more intensely than men do, which might help explain why women report painful conditions more often.

But the subjective nature of pain makes this a difficult call. For example, women may feel it's more socially acceptable to complain about pain than men, making them more willing to admit they're suffering. Or women may generally be more

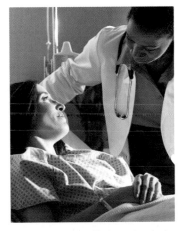

sensitive to suffering, both in themselves and others.

Yet research suggests there may be biological reasons that women experience more pain, perhaps due to factors that include genetics, hormones, biochemistry, and anatomy. Studies have found that certain types of prescription painkillers work better for women than for men (and vice versa), depending on how

the drugs bind to various receptors in the central nervous system. Not insignificantly, drugs that are apparently most effective for women, known as kappa-opioids, are less commonly prescribed than those that seem to work best for men.

Other gender differences related to treatment are even more striking. Despite the fact that women appear to suffer more, studies suggest that being female makes you more likely to be undertreated for pain. Pain specialists point to long-standing biases among doctors, who often assume that women exaggerate their pain. The reality may be different: On the basis of research, some experts contend that women are sensitive to such accusations and therefore may actually understate their pain.

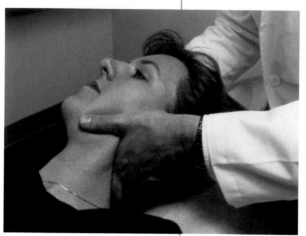

also trained in Western medicine and anatomy. Look for practitioners who are certified by the American Academy of Medical Acupuncture or a similar licensing organization.

■ **Chiropractor.** A doctor of chiropractic doesn't have as much medical training as a regular doctor, but may be able to help alleviate pain through manipulation. Be skeptical if a chiropractor says you need lots of X rays, and ask plenty of questions before undergoing treatment. For example, you should ask how long treatment sessions last, how many sessions you can expect to require, and whether the treatment itself will cause any discomfort or lasting aftereffects such as aching or stiffness.

■ **Massage therapist.** Often with offices in professional medical buildings, massage therapists can help relax muscles, limber up joints, and distract you from pain. Ask your doctor for a referral—and find out if you can talk to other patients who have used a particular therapist. Check that a therapist has been endorsed by a certifying authority such as the National Certification Board for Therapeutic Massage and Bodywork or the American Massage Therapy Association.

Dealing with Your Doctor

For flus, allergies, minor injuries, and routine exams— garden-variety reasons people see doctors—you might only see your physician for one or two visits, then not darken his door for long periods of time. But it's different when you're dealing with chronic pain. As with any lingering condition, you can expect to see your doctor more often than the average patient, making a smooth relationship all the more important.

While you and your doctor should remain open to your getting care elsewhere, your relationship is a potentially long-term partnership. But even long-term relationships often come down to a series of short-term encounters—in this case, with a person who is always under time constraints. That's why it's important to make the most of each visit with your doctor, especially at the beginning of your relationship.

HOW TO BEGIN

No matter how much medical history you have behind you, seeing a new doctor is a fresh start. He or she will certainly want to know everything in your chart, but shouldn't make any decisions based just on prior records. "A doctor needs to take time to do his own workup and find out what he thinks is wrong with you, not just spend 10 to 15 minutes based on earlier physicians' reports," says Mullin. In fact, studies find that 60 to 70 percent of the information a doctor needs comes from the patient's medical history—which includes a detailed discussion in which you explain your problems in your own words.

The pain assessment methods described in chapter 2 will help you and your doctor diagnose and understand the nature of your pain, as well as decide how to treat it. But during an initial visit, your doctor will want to know about the rest of your medical history as well.

Before you visit the doctor, be alert to symptoms you're experiencing other than pain, jotting down a record of when they occur, get better, or get worse. Be prepared to answer questions about health problems you've had previously, even

DR. WRONG: THE WARNING SIGNS

Nobody's perfect—your doctor included. But even when you're forgiving of personal faults, you don't have to accept substandard care or put up with a physician who makes you uncomfortable. Some early signs from your doctor that this may not be the start of a beautiful relationship:

Insensitivity. Some doctors want patients to be tough. But the point is how much he can help, not how much you can take.

Doubt. There should be no question in anyone's mind that your pain is real. If your doctor doesn't take your pain seriously, she won't take your treatment seriously either.

Low expectations. Your doctor may tell you there's nothing he can do. Take it at face value: There's nothing he can do. Someone else may be able to do more.

A deaf ear. Doctors treating pain have to be good listeners. If you get the feeling your physician doesn't want to hear about your pain, he's not likely to take any more interest in making you feel better.

Haughtiness. You have questions; maybe she has answers. But that does not make her the all-knowing expert or you the know-nothing dunce. Your doctor should never make you feel stupid or patronized.

QUESTIONS TO ASK YOUR DOCTOR

Starting a relationship with a doctor is like any other courtship: It involves a getting-to-know-you process in which there should be lots of give and take on both sides. Your doctor will certainly have plenty of questions for you. Here are a few you should have for him:

▶ What would be your strategy in treating my pain?

▶ What therapies do you start with, and what do you do next if they don't work?

▶ At what point do you start considering invasive or aggressive treatments such as nerve blocks, implanted pumps, or surgery?

▶ How many patients with my type of pain have you treated before?

▶ Do you feel opioids pose a danger of addiction? If so, would you hesitate to prescribe them if I needed them?

▶ If you're short on time, is there a nurse or other medical professional on your team who can answer my questions?

if they're not bothering you now or they seem trivial in retrospect. You can also expect your doctor to ask about your family history, so gather as much information as you can about problems that have affected your parents, siblings, or children—perhaps writing them down ahead of time so you don't forget to mention anything. In addition, your doctor will want to know what medications you're taking for any condition. This includes over-the-counter medicines and any herbal or nutritional supplements—all of which can interact with drugs your physician may want to prescribe.

MAKING THE MOST OF EACH VISIT

Once your doctor personally knows your history, you won't have to go through it every time you see him. But be sure to keep track of new symptoms or changes in your pain status between visits and bring this information to your next appointment. Without the need to take an extensive history, your doctor may reasonably expect follow-up visits to be shorter. But you can still accomplish a lot if you make smart use of the time you have. Some suggestions:

▶ **Get your priorities straight.** Before your appointment, make a list of everything you want to discuss. Rank the items in order of importance and share the list with your doctor at the beginning of the visit so you're both clear about your agenda. Don't put off asking disturbing or embarrassing questions to the end of the visit: Often these matters deserve placement at the top of your list and bringing them up as a "by the way" as you're heading out the door throws your entire visit off and may not gain you the careful attention you deserve.

▶ **Book the best appointment.** No matter how busy your doctor may be, some times of day are usually less frantic than others. Each doctor's office schedule is different, but early-morning appointments are often best because your physician is more likely to feel fresh and be running on time. In many offices, you're best off avoiding Mondays and Fridays: At the start of the week, patients often jam the schedule with problems that came up over the weekend, while at the end of the week, people rush to get exams and prescriptions before offices close. Check with the receptionist or nurse in charge of the calendar to learn your doctor's best times.

▶ **Write it down.** To help remember what your doctor tells you, bring along a pen and paper and take notes. If you don't understand everything your physician tells you, ask her to repeat the information so you're clear, and don't hesitate to bring up questions as you go. You don't have to get down every word: Focus mainly on issues that are best addressed in person (why she's switching you from one drug to another, for example), then ask for literature, websites, or organizations that can provide you with more detailed information you can delve into later. Another option: Bring a family member or friend who can listen objectively, provide support, and think of questions that may not occur to you. Have your companion take notes on the meeting so you can concentrate on interacting with your doctor.

HOW TO FIND A PAIN DOCTOR

Putting your care in the hands of a pain specialist first means finding the right doctor. Here are some ways to do it:

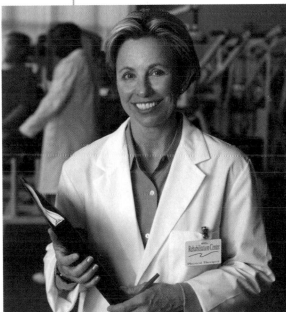

▶ **If you're part of a managed care plan**, ask for a list of pain specialists that are part of the doctor network from which you're allowed to choose.

▶ **Ask your regular doctor** to recommend a good pain specialist or clinic. But don't stop there. Also ask other doctors, nurses, technicians, pharmacists—anybody who might have an inside track on who really provides the best care.

▶ **If you're not part of a closed network of specialists,** call your area's largest local hospital and ask if it has a pain management program, or find out where the hospital refers pain patients. Another option: Call a local hospice program (regardless of whether you need hospice care) to ask which doctors they use or recommend for alleviating pain.

▶ **To learn all the options for your region**, log on to www.pain.com, which lists pain clinics and specialists for every state. You can also find state lists of accredited programs or doctors at the American Academy of Pain Management's site, www.aapainmanage.org, or by calling 209-533-9744.

Once you've narrowed your list of candidates, call their offices to ask if they're taking new patients and whether they accept your medical insurance. Find out if promising doctors have been certified by the American Board of Pain Medicine or belong to the American Pain Society.

Ask if you can interview promising candidates briefly on the phone or in person to get an idea of what they're like.

Should You Go to a Pain Center?

Going to a specialized pain center or clinic may not be your first choice in treating your pain. After all, many of the medications and therapies pain doctors use are available to other physicians as well. However, "just because there are a lot of tools in your garage doesn't mean you know how to fix your car," says Mullin. In fact, research suggests the expertise you gain with specialists may improve your odds of getting relief.

In one comparison involving 3,000 patients, only 17 percent of those who enrolled in pain clinics re-entered the hospital after a year, while 40 percent of patients who received just a single therapy did. Still, experts caution that it pays to be careful when considering specialized pain medicine because it's easy for any doctor (or alternative medicine practitioner) to hang a shingle for a pain clinic. "There are a lot of good private pain centers," says Mullin, "but some are not entirely kosher."

How can you decide if a pain clinic is right for you—or which you should choose? For starters, it helps to understand the different types of clinics you might encounter. Some are disease-oriented, offering treatments for specific conditions—most commonly arthritis, back pain, headaches, cancer, and chronic nerve and muscle disorders. Others emphasize specific types of treatment, such as medication, physical therapy, or various forms of alternative medicine such as chiropractic or acupuncture. In some instances, clinics are associated with hospitals, but many are independent, stand-alone centers. Some offer inpatient services in which you stay at the clinic during your treatment, while others provide outpatient care in which you come to the clinic only for appointments.

Which you choose depends first on the nature of your pain. If you know you suffer from a specific condition, then a specialty clinic for that condition may prove helpful. But in many cases, experts say chronic pain patients benefit most by choosing another option: going to a comprehensive pain center affiliated with a medical school or large hospital. At these multidisciplinary centers "we try to attack pain from several different angles at once," says Mullin.

Think of comprehensive centers as one-stop shops—offering a range of therapies that may include medication, physical therapy, osteopathy, psychological counseling, and even certain forms of alternative medicine. "I was apprehensive about going to a pain center at first because I thought they were just about providing pain medications," says Nicole Smith, whose pelvic joint disorder brought her to Spaulding Rehabilitation Hospital in Boston. "But they've taken a number of different approaches that together have helped me, and all the specialists there talk to each other, which doesn't always happen when you deal with doctors separately."

Whatever type of clinic you consider, Mullin and other experts advise weighing a number of factors when deciding where to entrust your care—and whether to stick with it once you begin. These include:

- **How doctors plan to treat you.** Find out which therapies the center offers on-site and which they tend to emphasize most. Be leery of pain centers that routinely steer patients into surgery or rely heavily on medications without a balance of other therapies. If you're interested in treatments the center doesn't offer, ask how—or if—doctors would provide them.
- **How much time doctors spend with you.** At many pain clinics, doctors take significantly more time diagnosing and treating problems than is typical in other medical settings. If you feel you're being rushed or given short shrift, it may be a

sign the clinic is more interested in business volume than helping patients.

■ **How well doctors explain things.** You should always have a clear understanding of why doctors prescribe a given therapy—and educating you about your pain should be a priority: Studies find that patients who have their treatment explained do better than those who are kept in the dark.

■ **Whether your treatment helps.** If you don't feel your pain has significantly improved after three to six months, you may want to try a different pain center.

Facing Financial Frustrations

As if chronic pain weren't distressing enough, it's often accompanied by a variety of financial concerns, ranging from loss of income due to disability to—especially—the challenge of paying for your care. If you have health insurance, it's likely you belong to a managed care plan such as an HMO. While these plans can be less expensive than traditional fee-for-service insurance, they often limit payment for pain medicine.

Pain doctors complain that insurance companies shortchange themselves by denying coverage of certain treatments. "A procedure such as spinal cord stimulation can be very expensive, but it can save money in the long run by reducing the need for surgery and ongoing doctor's visits," says Mullin. But don't assume your insurer won't pay: Every carrier is different—and you can sometimes persuade companies to pay for treatments they normally deny, particularly if other treatments have failed. Most companies have review boards or appeal processes that are not widely publicized.

To handle the challenges of paying for—or saving money on—your healthcare expenses, consider these steps:

▶ **Pore over the paperwork.** You must understand clearly what your policy actually provides. It may be mind-numbing, but you and your doctor can't talk to insurers about your coverage unless you go over your contract with a fine-tooth comb. The best time to do this is before you have services performed so you know in advance whether you'll be denied coverage—and whether you have cause to appeal that decision. If your policy is unclear about provisions for pain medicine, call your insurer and ask about the specific treatment you have in mind.

- ▶ **Call ahead.** The day before you see any pain care specialist, call to make sure the office received the referral from your primary-care physician and pre-authorization for your treatment from the insurance company By making sure all approvals are in place beforehand, you'll protect yourself from reimbursement problems after you've already paid for services.

- ▶ **Ferret out the formulary.** Most insurance plans have a list of approved medications that are covered by the policy—what's known as the formulary. Formulary drugs meet most patients' needs, but you can run into snags if your doctor prescribes a brand-name drug rather than a generic one, or steers you toward medications that are similar to—but more expensive than—those your insurer okays. If the drug your doctor prescribes isn't on the master list, ask him if an approved drug will work as well. If your doctor feels an unlisted drug is best, check with your insurer: You may be able to go off the formulary if your doctor can justify the exception or you agree to pay slightly more.

- ▶ **Make a case for your care.** Some insurance plans balk at paying for drugs usually prescribed for conditions other than what you're using them for—a common scenario with pain medicine. If your plan denies payment, have your doctor write a letter of appeal outlining why the drug is medically necessary. Bolster your case by finding studies that show the drug's safety and effectiveness.

The Pain-Relief Frontier

If pain medicine has advanced slowly over the long haul—morphine and aspirin are older than most of the patients who use them—scientists nevertheless have made remarkable progress in understanding and treating pain in recent years. Pain may still be vexing for patients and doctors alike, but doctors today have more options for dealing with discomfort than at any previous time in history.

"The message to carry into the future is that you don't have to suffer," says Frederick J. Goldstein, Ph.D., professor of clinical pharmacology at the Philadelphia College of Osteopathic Medicine. "You have a right to pain management and, while we may not be able to eliminate 100 percent of your pain, there's a lot we can do to make people comfortable."

This attitude may be one of the primary advances of twenty-first-century pain medicine, written into formal standards for pain management published by the Joint Commission on Accreditation of Healthcare Organizations in 1999 and now being implemented across the U.S. "If we simply put into place more of what we already know, patients will be much better off," Goldstein says.

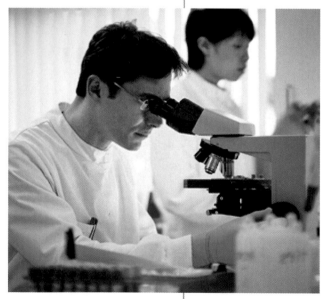

A DECADE OF PROGRESS

The new accreditation standards aren't the only initiative spurring progress in pain medicine. In late 2000, Congress declared the 10-year period starting in January 2001 as the Decade of Pain Control and Research, an unprecedented opportunity for pain management advocates to appeal for funding and legislation to help ease patient suffering.

A similar designation of the 1990s as the Decade of the Brain led to important advances in understanding brain chemistry, development, and function, which has also been helpful in unraveling the mysteries of pain. Now, for the years ahead, organizations like the American Pain Society, the American Pain Foundation, and the American Academy of Pain Medicine have formed a coalition to promote a variety of pain goals, including:

- More basic research into how pain works
- More studies on who experiences pain, what causes it, the prevalence of chronic versus acute pain, and how different forms of pain are treated
- More training for scientists interested in studying pain and its management
- Transferring research from labs and universities to clinical settings where it can help patients
- Doubling the funds the National Institutes of Health spends on pain research over the course of the decade
- Educating doctors on the importance of managing pain by designing curricula for medical schools, developing courses for annual meetings of specialty organizations, and creating a high-profile lecture series for the medical community
- Boosting public awareness through websites, public lectures, celebrity endorsements, and educational materials

"Scientists are focusing on pain in a way they never have before," says Dr. Mullin of the University of Michigan, Ann Arbor. "The entire medical community is awakening to the fact that pain is an important issue."

Where Research Is Going

In science, you can often get a hint of what lies ahead by looking back: The path to the future will be built on the bedrock of advances that have already taken place. For example, relatively recent NSAIDs such as naproxen have been improved upon by the new COX-2 anti-inflammatories—and more of the latter are in the pipeline. Meantime, as researchers inch forward in their understanding of pain's mechanisms, we get that much closer to newer, better drugs and therapies.

The complexity of pain gives researchers plenty of territory to explore—and research is continuing along every conceivable avenue, including investigations into pain's pathways through the nervous system, learning more about specific chronic conditions, and developing new medications.

BREAKING BIOLOGICAL BARRIERS

In the realm of "pure" research, scientists are coming to better understand the biological processes that contribute to pain, according to recent reports from the National Institute of Neurological Disorders and Stroke and numerous specialist organizations that deal with pain. Among the most recent developments:

■ **Pinpointing peptides.** These compounds, which help form building blocks for proteins, also play a role in pain responses that researchers are beginning to piece together. One peptide that appears related to pain is called substance P. Another is called tachykinins-neurokinin A. In experiments that hold promise for the development of new drugs, mice bred to lack a gene for these two peptides seemed to experience less pain, especially in the normally moderate-to-severe category. The promise is that such findings will point the way to drugs specifically designed to treat different grades of pain, particularly at the higher end of the intensity scale.

■ **Identifying a pain protein.** A similar study in mice by researchers at Johns Hopkins University finds that animals lacking a protein called PSD-93 tolerate pain better than regular mice. Physical exams of the mice may explain why: Areas of the spinal cord such as the dorsal horn that transport pain signals to the brain have naturally high concentrations of this protein. Researchers conclude that PSD-93 is essential for transmission of pain signals due to nerve injury, and that finding a way to block the protein provides a new potential target for preventing and treating chronic pain.

■ **Neutralizing needless pain.** In other research involving substance P, investigators have isolated a small group of nerve

---

DO REDHEADS NEED MORE RELIEF?

Every child understands that genetics are what make your eyes or hair a certain shade. But can such superficial expressions of our DNA affect how much pain we feel?

An intriguing study presented to the American Society of Anesthesiologists in late 2002 suggests that the answer may be yes. Researchers who gave anesthetic to women with various natural hair colors, then tested their response to painful stimuli, found that redheads needed about 20 percent more anesthesia than women with dark or blond hair. The study was the first to suggest that visible genetic traits may be related to pain sensitivity—potentially important, for example, when people are put under for surgery.

One explanation for the redhead response is that a cell receptor that brightly pigmented people lack may be tied to a hormone that boosts pain perception in the brain. The hair-color finding may not only have practical importance when it comes to using anesthesia, but may help scientists understand just how anesthetic gases make people lose consciousness and become impervious to pain—basic mechanisms that are still largely mysterious.

cells in the spinal cord that appear critical to ferrying chronic pain signals. Using substance P receptors as a way to gain access to these neurons, scientists have been able to kill the cells with a chemical in animals. Result: Within days, animals receiving the neuron-killing mix no longer showed signs of chronic pain. Even more remarkable, the animals were still able to feel acute, or "healthy," pain necessary to avoid harm from injury. The hope is that researchers may be able to develop treatments that have similarly specific effects in people.

■ **Attacking arthritis.** In recent papers for the American College of Rheumatology, researchers have reported new ways to reduce the body's levels of tumor necrosis factor (TNF), a natural protein that causes joint inflammation and damage in people with rheumatoid arthritis (RA). Doing so can improve symptoms of the disease, and the new methods may provide alternatives to etanercept (Enbrel), an expensive new "designer drug" for RA that also lowers TNF levels. In a study of one treatment, about two-thirds of patients showed significant improvement after getting a series of injections of a TNF antibody called adalimumab, which binds to TNF and removes it from the body. Similar results were seen in a three-month trial of another injected anti-TNF therapy, with improvement in some cases kicking in within a week. In both studies, treatments were effective even with patients who had poor luck with other types of therapy for the disease.

JUMPING ON GENETICS

You may not think of pain as a genetically determined problem, but rapidly expanding insights into the body's master code are helping scientists understand the underlying basis for some forms of pain, and may eventually lead to new treatments. Among the developments:

■ **Forecasting neuropathy.** In a study presented to the American Neurological Association in late 2002, scientists at Duke University found that variations in a gene implicated in heart disease and Alzheimer's disease may also help predict the severity of peripheral neuropathy. Common in people with diabetes, peripheral neuropathy occurs when nerves in the body's outlying areas, such as the feet, become damaged and cause a variety of sensations, including numbness, cramps, or burning pain. Patients with the high-risk genetic variation were likely to develop neuropathy and related complications much earlier than other at-risk people, the researchers reported. Identifying highest-risk patients early may help guide treatment and (in the case of diabetes) lifestyle-based steps to prevent neuropathy, staving off complications that include pain, amputation, and even premature death.

■ **Tailoring treatment.** The promise of much genetically based medicine in the future is to tailor treatment to patients' individual genetic makeup. In the case of pain, for example, scientists have found that some people who don't respond to codeine lack a liver enzyme called CYP2D6, which helps convert codeine into morphine. Researchers are now looking into the role the enzyme plays in pain relief, and may eventually be able to better design treatments for people with deficiencies.

FINE-TUNING PHARMACEUTICALS

Drug companies have plenty of incentive to find new solutions to the challenges of chronic pain: The scope of the problem is large, and new pain-relief standards for healthcare facilities potentially make the market even bigger.

Among the challenges are designing clinical trials that take into account the highly individual nature of discomfort and the wide variety of factors that can affect how people respond to pain—and its treatment. But while "magic bullets" may be few and far between, we can expect to see incremental breakthroughs as drug therapies continue to be refined. Some of what's on the horizon:

■ **Even better NSAIDs.** In the late 1990s, COX-2 drugs were hailed as breakthroughs because they dulled pain while damaging the stomach less than older nonsteroidal anti-inflammatories. Research suggests, however, that COX-2s may raise heart health risks for certain people. Now a new anti-inflammatory, finishing up clinical trials in Europe, appears to be an even better option. At a conference in Sweden in 2002, researchers said the new drug, called licofelone, blocks enzymes that produce inflammation-causing prostaglandins (as do other NSAIDs), but is gentle on the stomach and appears not to raise the risk of complications like blood clots. Further trials and a formal request to license the drug are to be completed as soon as possible.

■ **Fewer side effects.** One of the major goals in pain medication is to develop drugs that are as powerful and effective as opioids already available, but have fewer side effects such as nausea and sedation—not to mention tolerance and dependence. According to the National Institute of Neurological Disorders and Stroke, studies have identified a number of factors that contribute to the development of tolerance. Further research should eventually lead to opioids that patients can take in lower doses or that are formulated or packaged with opioid antagonists to prevent illicit use and abuse.

■ **New delivery techniques.** Drug developers are also looking at ways to reduce the need for potent pain medications by using existing analgesics in new ways. For example, a recent study found that a system delivering non-narcotic numbing medication directly into an incision site after open heart or foot and ankle surgery reduced the need for post-op opioids by more than 60 percent. Called the ON-Q Post-Op Pain Relief System, the delivery method also cut the amount of time patients spent in the hospital by almost a third.

THE ROAD AHEAD

Behind the scenes, researchers are also debating basic questions of how doctors might best apply new knowledge as it's obtained. As we learn more about how pain works, will we be able to treat pain based on what's specifically causing it (an approach known as mechanism-based treatment), or should we concentrate on developing medications that work well for the broadest possible range of conditions? Which approach is most feasible? What will ultimately be best for patients? Is research money being funneled into the disciplines that are best able to treat the most common kinds of pain? These are the kinds of questions currently being debated in the pain management field. The fact that such debates are taking place is a sign of hope: No matter what decisions are made, progress in pain management continues with lots of attention, and patients will ultimately be better able to subdue their suffering.

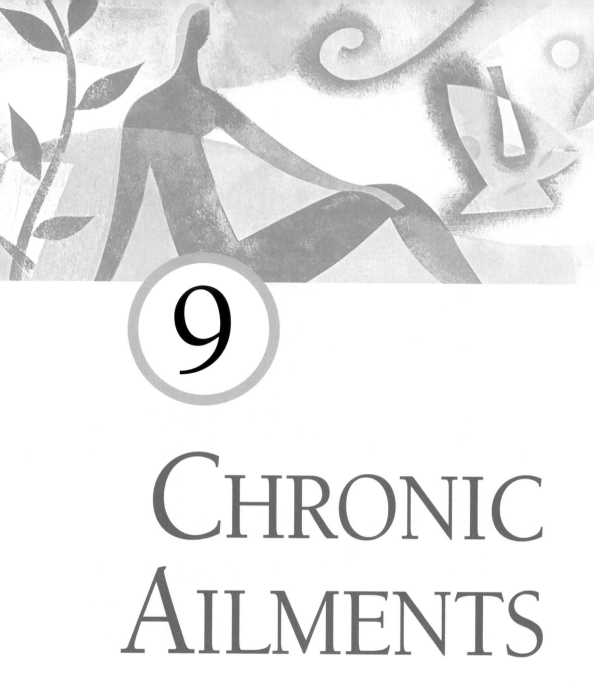

9

CHRONIC AILMENTS

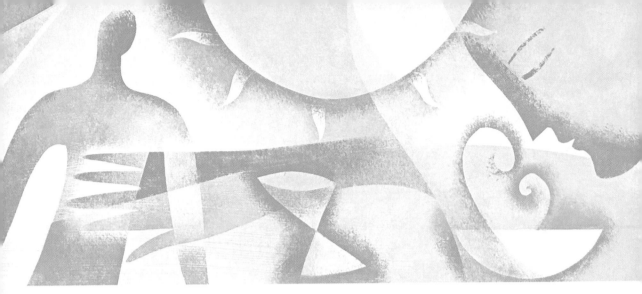

- Arthritis

- Back Pain

- Cancer Pain

- Carpal Tunnel Syndrome

- Central Pain Syndrome
  (Thalamic Syndrome)

- Chronic Fatigue Syndrome

- Complex Region Pain Syndrome

- Endometriosis

- Fibromyalgia

- Interstitial Cystitis

- Irritable Bowel Syndrome

- Migraine and other Headaches

- Neck Pain

- Peptic Ulcer

- Peripheral Neuropathy

- Postherpetic Neuralgia

- Premenstrual Syndrome

- Rheumatoid Arthritis

- Temporomandibular Joint
  Disorder

- Trigeminal Neuralgia

I f you're afflicted with the pain and stiffness of arthritis, you've got plenty of company. Arthritis is emerging as a leading cause of disability in the United States. But having the condition needn't mean endless pain or inactivity. You have a lot of flexibility when it comes to choosing forms of relief. Your anti-arthritis program should include home remedies and medications for immediate soothing of pain, as well as a long-term foundation of healthy eating and exercise to help protect and strengthen your joints.

Understanding the Pain

By far the most common form of arthritis is osteoarthritis (OA), which affects more than 36 million Americans. (For information on the second most common form, rheumatoid arthritis, see page 244.) Sometimes called "wear and tear" arthritis, OA occurs when decades of use causes cartilage—the shock-absorbing material between the joints—to break down. The more joints degenerate, the less smoothly they move, until eventually, exposed bones rub together, triggering pain and stiffness that limits movement, especially in hard-working joints such as the knees, hips, hands, feet, and spine. If you have OA, you'll usually find the afflicted joint feels stiffest the first 5 to 10 minutes after rising in the morning, and may hurt or swell during and after use, but pain improves with rest. Sometimes small growths called bone spurs can form around the outer edges of bones, pinching nerves or poking joints, which causes even more pain and tenderness.

OA often begins during midlife, around age 45, but many people don't notice symptoms until they reach their 60s. Older women are especially vulnerable, with women over 65 twice as likely to develop OA of the knee as elderly men. But while OA is almost inevitable with advanced age, some factors do make you more susceptible or can make the condition worse once you have it. These include:

INSTANT ACTION

- Elevate a swollen joint and apply an ice pack.

- Dissolve pain with moist heat or a tingling ointment.

- Swallow a pain reliever such as acetaminophen or an NSAID.

- Reduce stress on painful, often-used joints with a splint, cane, shoe wedges, or other physical devices.

- Meditate or practice deep breathing to help cope with a pain flare-up.

➤ Obesity, because excess weight puts added stress on joints

➤ Damaging joints during physical labor or strenuous sports

➤ Lack of exercise (moderate physical activity helps keep joints flexible and muscles strong)

➤ Past injury

➤ Family history

SELF-CARE STRATEGIES

Heat. The moist heat of a hot bath or shower eases pain and stiffness of OA. In lieu of a full-body treatment, hold a hot-water bottle, heating pad, or hot pack on the aching area. Heat can be especially soothing when alternated with contrasting treatments of cold. One way to do it: Soak the aching joint in warm water for 10 minutes, then cold water for one minute. Continue this process for about half an hour, ending with a warm dunk. Cold alone works best for inflamed joints—a characteristic of rheumatoid arthritis, but not OA.

Hot wax. If you want to take heat relief to the next level, indulge in a paraffin bath: Coat hands or feet with the hot, waxy substance and leave on while it cools, trapping in heat. Many day spas offer hot-wax treatments, or you can find do-it-yourself kits at medical-supply firms or drugstores.

Helpful devices. Osteoarthritis is one of a handful of chronically painful conditions that can be managed with the help of simple devices designed to ease strain on aching joints. These include collars, splints, braces, crutches, canes, grip devices, orthopedic shoes, and heel wedges. Ask a physical or occupational therapist for a catalog of products, check with your local pharmacy or medical supply store, or use an Internet search engine to find online suppliers. Check with your doctor to make sure that the products you are considering are right for your condition.

Weight loss. For long-term relief from arthritis pain, shedding pounds can take strain off your joints, reducing pain and increasing mobility. A little loss goes a long way: Each pound you drop eases the load on the knee by three to five pounds while walking—which means a 10-pound loss could relieve weight-bearing joints of 30 to 50 pounds of added stress.

Exercise. Don't let joint pain keep you sidelined: To lose

CHECKLIST FOR RELIEF

✔ Self-Care Strategies

Heat treatment	p. 88
Contrast baths	p. 88
Joint-protecting devices	
Drop pounds if overweight	p.148
Aerobic exercise	p.104
Strengthening exercises	p.106
Stretching exercises	p. 92

✔ Medical Measures

Pain-relieving ointments	p. 49
Acetaminophen	p. 44
NSAIDs	p. 41
Tramadol	p. 50
Other opioids	p. 45
Corticosteroid injections	p. 44
Injected hyaluronic acid	p.175
Surgery	

✔ Complementary Options

Glucosamine and chondroitin sulfate	p.123
Yoga	p. 96
T'ai chi	p. 97
Meditation	p. 78
Imagery	p. 74
Acupuncture	p.113

weight, you have to both cut the number of calories you consume and burn more through exercise—another key part of arthritis management. Bonus benefit: According to the National Institute of Arthritis and Musculoskeletal and Skin Diseases, regular activity can sometimes help decrease pain enough to delay the need for pain-relieving drugs. In addition, exercise increases flexibility, improves mood, and promotes general health. Although you should ask your doctor or physical therapist to help design the best exercise program for you, most people can benefit from a program that includes aerobic exercises such as walking and swimming, along with stretching exercises to increase flexibility and resistance training to increase strength.

MEDICAL MEASURES

Topical pain-tamers. Try rubbing out OA pain with topical pain relievers that contain camphor, menthol, or other counter-irritants that feel cool or warm—sensations that can mask the underlying pain. Examples include Arthricare Double Ice, Aspercreme, Ben Gay, Eucalyptamint, Icy Hot, Sportscreme, or topical products containing capsaicin, a pain-relieving substance derived from hot chili peppers, such as Capzasin-P and Zostrix.

First-line analgesics. For more systemic relief, the first defense against OA is often over-the-counter acetaminophen (Tylenol), which has been shown to be both safe and effective. For persistent pain or swelling, try an OTC nonsteroidal anti-inflammatory drug (NSAID) such as aspirin, ibuprofen, or naproxen-—or move on to prescription COX-2 drugs such as Celebrex, Vioxx, and Bextra if regular NSAIDs upset your stomach. Osteoarthritis patients often find that some NSAIDs work better for them than others, so don't give up on all NSAIDs if one product doesn't work well.

Stronger painkillers. Moderate to severe pain may require

BE CAUTIOUS ABOUT SURGERY

Successful surgery may get you back in the swing if you've been sidelined by pain, but keep in mind that all surgery poses risks and even this last resort for arthritis treatment may not be a real solution. For example, in a new study, OA patients who underwent knee arthroscopy—a minimally invasive form of joint repair—fared no better than those who got a placebo procedure in which knife nicks in the knee falsely suggested surgery was done. "Twenty to forty percent of patients will get better because they expect to," says Gary S. Firestein, M.D., chief of the division of rheumatology, allergy, and immunology at the University of California in San Diego. "The more important-sounding, invasive, and aggressive the treatment, the greater the placebo effect." If a doctor suggests surgery, be sure to get a second opinion.

a step up to stronger drugs. Opioids are one option. Your doctor may start you on tramadol (Ultram), which binds less potently to opioid receptors in the nervous system. It appears to be particularly beneficial for OA sufferers, while causing relatively fewer side effects than more powerful opioids.

Steroid injections. If painkilling pills don't relieve intense pain or inflammation, your doctor may suggest corticosteroids, which may be injected into joints such as knees two or three times a year to gain you about a three-week reprieve from discomfort. Don't expect ongoing treatment with steroids: Because of concern about side effects such as ulcers and weight gain, doctors generally prescribe them only for short periods at a time.

Possible procedures. When drugs and less drastic measures fail to control arthritis pain, it may be time to turn to an orthopedic surgeon. Joint-saving operations include:

➤**Arthroplasty**, or total joint replacement. Substituting an artificial joint for the damaged one is most commonly done in hips and knees, but replacements can also restore mobility to shoulders, elbows, wrists, and fingers.

➤**Arthroscopy**, or removing pieces of bone and damaged cartilage.

➤**Osteotomy**, or realigning the joint.

➤**Synovectomy**, or removing the synovial membrane that surrounds the joint.

A SHOT AT PAIN RELIEF

Just as a squirt of oil makes tight, squeaky machine parts work more smoothly, a shot of **hyaluronic acid** (Hyalgan, Synvisc), a natural fluid found in freely moving joints, may help stiff, creaky knees move more easily and with less pain. After three to five treatments, weekly injections of the jelly-like substance may provide up to six months of pain relief from osteoarthritis of the knees.

COMPLEMENTARY OPTIONS

With arthritis affecting so many people, an inevitably wide array of unconventional treatments has cropped up, from copper jewelry costing just a few dollars to high-tech pulsed electromagnetic therapy (which bathes the body with electromagnetic fields) costing $1,800 a session. "Be very wary of reported cures and treatments unless they've been appropriately studied—and few have been," says Gary S. Firestein, M.D., chief of the division of rheumatology, allergy, and immunology at the University of California in San Diego. Alternative therapies should complement, not replace, a medical pain-control program.

READY RESOURCES

Arthritis Foundation
P.O. Box 7669
Atlanta, GA 30357-0669
Phone: 800-283-7800
Website: www.arthritis.org

**National Institute of
Arthritis and Musculoskeletal
and Skin Diseases**
National Institutes of Health
One AMS Circle
Bethesda, MD 20892-3675
Phone: 877-226-4267
Fax: 301-718-6366
Website: www.niams.nih.gov

Natural joint builders. Among the hottest alternative treatments on the market for joint pain are glucosamine and chondroitin sulfate. These over-the-counter supplements are designed to replicate joint-protecting substances found naturally in the body. In Europe, glucosamine and chondroitin sulfate have been used to treat OA for more than 10 years, and preliminary studies suggest that the supplements may indeed help repair and maintain cartilage, easing pain as well as or better than NSAIDs—but with few side effects. A clinical trial supported by the National Institutes of Health (NIH) is under way to determine if either compound—or a combination of the two—offers long-lasting symptom relief.

Acupuncture. Some NIH studies have been done on acupuncture. Early findings suggest it may help reduce pain and improve function in patients with OA of the knee.

Mental methods. On the mind/body front, methods such as meditation, imagery, and deep breathing can help you better cope with pain—and they cost nothing (apart from training sessions) and have no side effects. "Moving meditation" techniques such as yoga and t'ai chi do double duty by gently working the body while occupying the mind.

OTHER TYPES OF ARTHRITIS

Though osteoarthritis and rheumatoid arthritis account for most cases, arthritis (which means "joint inflammation" in Latin) isn't a single condition, but a group of more than 100 different diseases that cause movement-limiting pain, stiffness, and swelling in the joints and connective tissues. Here are some of the other varieties:

- **ARTHRITIC INFECTIONS:** stiff, painful joints following a bacterial infection such as Lyme disease, gonorrhea, or a staphylococcal infection
- **ANKYLOSING SPONDYLITIS:** stiff, painful back from inflamed spinal joints, tendons, and ligaments; most common in men
- **GOUT:** intense pain and swelling in a single foot joint, usually the big toe; most common in older men
- **LUPUS:** aching joints all over the body; rash; may affect internal organs; most common in young women
- **PSEUDOGOUT:** painful, swollen joint in the knee, wrist, or ankle
- **PSORIATIC ARTHRITIS:** red, scaly rash as well as joint inflammation, usually in the fingers, toes, and knees
- **REACTIVE ARTHRITIS:** aching joints in arms and legs; heel pain; urinary tract discharge; eye inflammation; rash
- **SCLERODERMA:** tight, hardened skin; systemic type may affect several organs
- **SJÖGREN'S SYNDROME:** dry mouth and eyes from inflamed tear and saliva glands

At some point, almost everyone gets a backache. It hurts, you're miserable—but eventually the problem, like the strain that probably caused it, goes away. Then there is chronic back pain, when something is physically wrong with your spine or back that may not be easily identified or fixed, and the torment goes on for weeks, months, years. Such pain can sap you of energy and spirit if you let it— but you don't have to. Never before have there been so many medicines, low-tech physical therapies, and lifestyle tools to minimize recurrent back pain. With enough persistence and experimenting, most people with chronic back pain can regain their active lives with few, if any, constraints.

Understanding the Pain

Consisting of an S-shaped stack of 24 bones called vertebrae that run from the neck to the lower back, the spine provides the body with stability (for standing straight) and flexibility (for moving every which way). It also holds the spinal cord—including the nerve network that transmits both sensory and motor impulses between the brain and the body. Given its complexity, it's not surprising the back and its various components are vulnerable to a variety of insults (at least some of which hit four of five adults at some point in life). These problems include strained muscles, sprained ligaments, ruptured disks, and pinched nerves.

It's not always clear what causes these back problems to occur. "Sixty percent of the time, people who develop back pain don't really know why," says Richard A. Deyo, M.D., M.P.H., professor of medicine and health services at the University of Washington in Seattle. But there are plenty of possibilities:

Misuse. In many cases, improperly bending, twisting, or lifting puts too much strain on muscles, tendons, and ligaments,

INSTANT ACTION

■ Take an over-the-counter analgesic such as acetaminophen, aspirin, ibuprofen, or naproxen sodium, first-line mainstays of medical treatment.

■ If pain is related to a muscle strain, apply an ice pack to reduce swelling.

■ If pain is without swelling, soak in a warm bath or apply a heating pad to increase blood circulation.

■ For short-term relief, lie down. Put pillows under your knees to keep them elevated, easing muscle strain on the lower back.

■ Change high heels for flat- or low-heeled shoes: High heels put added strain on the lower back.

■ Practice good posture both standing and sitting.

BACK PAIN
Ailments

especially in the curve of the lower back or at the base of the neck. Pain may arise suddenly from, for example, a sharp twist to the side, or develop slowly, perhaps after years of slouching behind a desk or toting a heavy shoulder bag. Extremes of activity—either sitting around too much at home and work or overdoing strenuous exercise—put you at higher risk of problems, as does obesity because of the extra load excess weight places on the backbone.

Disk problems. Sometimes normal wear and tear or unusual strain can cause a disk (the spongy cushion between vertebrae) to bulge and rupture, putting pressure on spinal-column nerves. Known as a herniated disk, this can cause mild discomfort to severe pain, depending on whether the disk simply slips slightly out of place or pushes through and presses on neighboring nerves and structures. One common example: A herniated disk may pinch or squeeze the roots of the sciatic nerve, causing pain to shoot from the buttock and down the leg, a condition known as sciatica.

Compression fractures. The bone loss that occurs with age sometimes causes vertebrae to collapse onto each other (often apparent as a deformity known as dowager's hump).

Scoliosis. This abnormal curvature of the spine can start in childhood or adolescence.

Chronic health problems. Back pain can be part of a range of conditions affecting the spine, including osteoarthritis, a degenerative joint condition; rheumatoid arthritis, an autoimmune disorder; ankylosing spondylitis, in which the vertebrae fuse together; and fibromyalgia, which causes musculoskeletal pain. Illnesses such as kidney, gynecological, and intestinal diseases can also bring on aching backs.

SELF-CARE STRATEGIES

Ice and heat. Start by using a chilling ice pack (or even a bag of frozen vegetables), which can reduce soreness and swelling, especially if you've suffered an injury. Apply the cold for 15 to 20 minutes at a time (taking care not to freeze the skin), repeating every two hours or so during waking hours. After a couple of days, when any swelling should have subsided, switch to a heating pad or hot-water bottle to help muscles relax and loosen up, or take a long soak in a steamy bath for the added benefit of soothing stimulation from water.

Exercise. You'll be tempted to ease off your normal routine while in pain, but it's important to keep moving as much as possible: Long-term bed rest, once the standard treatment for back pain, may actually delay recovery by weakening muscles and bones. It's sensible to avoid movements that aggravate pain, and a day or two of rest may be appropriate following a flare-up, but after that, try easing back into everyday life. Consult your doctor about what activities you should limit—or get more of. For example, regular exercise may help reduce back pain as well as cut down on recurrent episodes. Aerobic workouts such as walking, biking, and swimming (a low-impact exercise that's especially easy on the back) help lower-back muscles function better, while stretching exercises promote flexibility. Resistance training helps strengthen the muscles that support and protect your spine

Posture. Your mother's healthy advice helps save your back: Keep your posture straight and upright while standing and sitting, to keep your spine in proper alignment. Women with back pain should give up high heels, which put added strain on the lower back.

Weight control. Extra pounds put pressure on the back. Eat a healthy, low-fat, low-calorie diet to keep unnecessary weight from burdening your back.

Back-friendly furniture. Sit on upright chairs (like dining room chairs); they encourage better posture than low, soft chairs and are easier to get out of. A plywood board under your bed may make you sleep more comfortably; plywood boards under your sofa seat pillows will give you more support when you sit there.

Back-friendly products. A wide range of products designed to take strain off the back, support the spine, or promote good posture are available from medical supply stores, catalogs and websites. For example, at www.backworks.com, one

FINE-TUNING FUSION

Traditionally, spinal fusion calls for one surgery to harvest bone from the pelvis, followed by another operation to weld together vertebrae with the harvested bone and metal rods.

Now, with a new bone-grafting device, patients who need the surgery may get by with just one operation instead of two. The Infuse Bone Graft was recently approved by the Food and Drug Administration. The cage-like device, implanted between the affected vertebrae, contains a genetically engineered protein that stimulates bone growth, so there's no need to use bone from the hip. Just how well this works remains to be seen, however. "At this point, it's unclear whether this technique will be as effective as older methods," says Richard A. Deyo, M.D., professor of medicine at the University of Washington.

of many sites, you'll find ergonomic chairs, pads and supports for chairs and car seats, special pillows and other sleep aids, self-massage tools, hot packs, and belts or braces that shore up the spine, among other products.

MEDICAL MEASURES

Pain relievers. Back pain generally eases with the help of OTC nonsteroidal anti-inflammatory drugs (NSAIDs), such as aspirin, ibuprofen (Advil, Motrin, and Nuprin) or naproxen sodium (Aleve). The cooling or warming effects of topical creams such as Ben Gay and Icy Heat can also provide comfort by stimulating nerves with sensations that help mask pain.

If these methods don't provide adequate relief, your doctor may reach for more potent painkillers such as an opioid (often codeine or tramadol). Depending on the nature of your pain, your doctor may also try corticosteroid injections to relieve severe pain and inflammation. A muscle relaxant such as methocarbamol or cyclobenzaprine (which work on the nervous system to make muscles less tight) may be used for a few days, but generally no longer because of unpleasant side effects such as nausea, disorientation, and drowsiness.

Physical therapy. A physical therapist will use ultrasound (high-frequency sound waves) to increase circulation and reduce inflation, hot and cold packs, as well as hydrotherapy for back pain. If pain stems from a compressed nerve, as it does in sciatica, the physical therapist may use transcutaneous electrical nerve stimulation (TENS) to help block nerve signals from reaching the brain. The therapist tapes electrodes near the source of the pain, and they carry a mild current to the affected area. For ongoing treatment, patients often learn to use TENS units on their own.

Possible procedures. Be sure to explore all your options before agreeing to surgery. Although back operations are common in the United States, only 2 percent of people with pain actually require surgery, according to the federal Agency for Healthcare Research and Quality (AHRQ). "Almost all back surgery is elective, but it's costly and poses risks of its own," says Deyo. "Many experts believe too much is being done in this country." (Twice as many back surgeries are performed in the

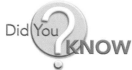

Did You KNOW

Aching backs aren't for adults only: Schoolchildren who haul over-loaded backpacks also complain of pain. Heavy bags strain the spine and shoulder, causing muscle fatigue and strain—especially when a kid slings on a pack using just one strap. Toting excessive weight could also lead to poor posture or constant slouching—habits that can cause bad backs. The American Academy of Orthopaedic Surgeons suggests that kids carry packs with wide, padded straps—and use both straps, along with a hip strap for especially heavy loads. The heaviest items should be placed closest to the back for better weight distribution.

U.S. as in any other developed country.) Get a second—or third—opinion when exploring even the most common surgeries. These include:

➤ **Spinal fusion,** which joins two vertebrae with metal implants, often to treat degenerative joint disease

➤ **Laminectomy,** in which doctors remove a portion of the bone overlaying the spinal cord

➤ **Diskectomy,** in which doctors remove disk fragments that bulge into the spinal canal or press on nerve roots

➤ **Foraminotomy,** in which doctors remove bone to enlarge the openings for nerve roots

➤ **Rhizotomy,** which involves severing a nerve so it stops sending pain signals to the brain

COMPLEMENTARY OPTIONS

Spinal manipulation. The AHRQ reports that spinal manipulation by a chiropractor or osteopath, who manipulates or massages the back to relieve pain and restore function, is effective for some patients. Studies suggest that these methods work as well as some other forms of physical therapy for low-back pain, although they may cost more if your insurance doesn't pay for your sessions. Chiropractors average 10 visits per episode of pain.

Acupuncture. Some doctors also advise acupuncture for patients who aren't relieved by mainstream measures, but evidence that acupuncture relieves back pain remains conflicting or ambiguous, says Dr. Deyo.

Massage. With your doctor's consent, you may benefit from Swedish massage in addition to other back pain therapies. Its stroking movements relax the tensed muscles around the painful area.. Rolfing and other deep massage techniques, however, can further damage a herniated disk and should be avoided.

LIFTING 101

Even when your spine's feeling fine again, it's important to prevent future pain by using proper form for everyday activities. Don't simply bend and stretch to lift a heavy item; that puts undue stress on the back. Instead, lift with your legs to spare the back and prevent injury:

(1) Squat down bending your legs, not your waist.

(2) Grasp the object directly in front of you, keeping your back straight.

(3) Stand straight up again, using your legs to lift and holding the load close to your body.

There may not be a cure for cancer yet, but years of diligent research have given us improved screenings to detect disease earlier (when cancer is most easily treated) and potent therapies that allow more patients to live longer—often cancer-free. And while cancer pain is still often undertreated, according to a statement that emerged from a 2002 National Institutes of Health conference on symptom management in cancer, many effective strategies for relief are readily available. In fact, 9 out of 10 people with cancer should be able to control pain enough to be physically comfortable—provided healthcare teams design effective, personal pain management plans.

INSTANT ACTION

■ Make clear to your doctor that you expect pain to be controlled aggressively.

■ Take your medicine as directed; trying to tough it out can make the pain worse and harder to control.

■ Get a pain assessment that puts a number on your discomfort so you and your doctors share an understanding of what you're going through.

■ Start a pain diary to gauge the effects of whatever treatment methods you try.

■ Try NSAIDs to start, but ask your doctor for stronger drugs if you feel they're necessary.

■ Practice mind/body techniques such as imagery, relaxation, and meditation to take better control of your pain.

Understanding the Pain

The more than 100 types of cancer affect nearly every part of the body, including the skin and all that lies beneath it: organs and glands (carcinoma), the lymphatic system (lymphoma), blood (leukemia), and bone, muscle, and cartilage (sarcoma). All involve trouble with cells, which normally divide and replace themselves in a controlled manner, but with cancer multiply with abandon, forming a mass, or tumor. Benign, non-cancerous tumors stop growing or grow very slowly—but malignant, cancerous tumors continue to enlarge, elbowing out healthy cells, damaging tissues, invading neighboring organs, and sometimes spreading throughout the body via the bloodstream.

Whatever their causes and consequences, most cancers have a common denominator in pain, with sharp, aching, burning, or throbbing pains arising as tumors spread into tissues, organs, or bone; press on nerves; or block hollow structures such as blood vessels or parts of the digestive system. Treatment for cancer can exacerbate the situation: Chemotherapy, radiotherapy, and surgery help rid the body of the cancer that's causing the discomfort, but the procedures themselves can cause pain: Chemotherapy may cause mouth sores, peripheral neuropathy (damage to the peripheral nerves), and gastrointestinal problems; radiation can irritate the skin and other organs; and surgery inevitably produces post-operative pain and scarring.

Pain with cancer is common, but not everyone suffers to the same degree. In fact, only about 25 percent of newly diagnosed patients experience pain, though discomfort generally grows with the tumor. About one-third of patients undergoing treatment, and two-thirds of those with advanced disease, experience acute, chronic, or worse-than-usual breakthrough pain. For those who are suffering, it's important to realize that almost all cancer pain can be successfully managed.

SELF-CARE STRATEGIES

Cancer is a beast with many heads; how you fight it—and the pain it causes—depends on the nature of the disease that's attacking. Your doctor can advise you on what to expect during the course of your illness and how the treatments you receive may affect you. But the same arsenal of weapons is available to any patient, beginning with simple treatments and comforting measures you can employ at home.

Temperature tinkering. Applying heat with a hot pack, heating pad, or hot-water bottle can soothe sore muscles and bone pain, while applying cold with a frozen gel pack (available at most drugstores), ice pack, or towel-wrapped ice cubes can numb the painful area. According to the National Cancer Institute (NCI), some cancer patients find that cold relieves pain faster and longer, though many people favor heat. The best approach may be to alternate heat and cold. For another approach try menthol creams and gels, which produce a soothing sensation that distracts from pain, sometimes for hours.

Skin stimulation. The NCI also recommends stimulating the skin using massage or even simple pressure from the heel of your hand, fingertips, knuckles, or thumbs. Aim to apply firm pressure on or around the painful area—as long as you don't cause more pain. Pressing for up to one minute can relieve pain for as long as several hours in some cases.

CHECKLIST FOR RELIEF

✔ **Self-Care Strategies**

Heat/cold treatments	p. 88
Topical ointments	p. 49
Massage	p.100
Pressure	
Vibration	
Exercise	p.103

✔ **Medical Measures**

Acetaminophen	p. 44
NSAIDs	p. 41
Weak opioids	p. 48
Strong opioids	p. 48
Antidepressants	p.136
Anticonvulsants	p. 49
Corticosteroids	p. 44
Nerve blocks	p. 55
Injection therapies	p. 54
Neurosurgery	p. 56

✔ **Complementary Options**

Acupuncture	p.113
TENS	p.102
Breathing exercises	p. 71
Relaxation therapy	p. 76
Visualization	p. 74
Meditation	p. 78
Touch therapies	p. 74

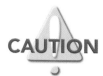

CAUTION

Consult your doctor about using even simple techniques that stimulate the skin—including heat and cold, pressure, and vibration: They may not be advisable during chemotherapy or radiation therapy. The National Cancer Institute also warns that you should avoid heat or cold treatments in areas treated with radiation for six months after the therapy has ended.

Exercise. The rigors of cancer treatment and pain can take the stuffing out of anybody, but it's a good idea to keep as active as possible. In addition to preventing loss of physical function, aerobic exercises such as walking and swimming appear to help control nausea from chemotherapy. Don't push yourself beyond what you can comfortably tolerate, however, and check with your doctor about what activities are best for you.

Practical help. Vibrating painful areas using battery-operated massage devices available in most pharmacies can provide temporary relief for many patients, according to the NCI. But you can also gain comfort from simpler aids, especially if illness and pain keep you from getting up. For example, pillows and foam rolls placed beneath the knees, lower back, and head offer extra relief in bed. If necessary, ask your doctor about splints, supports, and braces that can help reduce movement-related pain.

MEDICAL MEASURES

Generally, cancer-pain treatment follows a ladder approach recommended by the World Health Organization (WHO), in which you step up to increasingly stronger medications or drug combinations as pain continues to persist.

Non-opioids. Familiar over-the-counter pain relievers are the first step for mild pain, such as in bone or muscle. These include acetaminophen (Tylenol) and nonsteroidal anti-inflammatory drugs (NSAIDs) such as ibuprofen (Advil, Motrin, and Nuprin) and naproxen (Aleve). Treatment usually starts with low doses, which may be gradually increased up to a maximum "ceiling" dose beyond which these drugs have no greater effect. At that point, you take another step up the ladder, to opioids.

LICKING BREAKTHROUGH PAIN

A medicinal lollipop containing the opioid fentanyl (p.57) appears especially effective for reducing breakthrough pain in cancer patients. A 2001 study in the *Journal of Pain Management* found that cancer patients who used the lollipop for more than a year reported it to be 90 percent effective at controlling breakthrough pain; less than a third needed to increase the dose over time.

Opioids. Mild to moderate pain that's not relieved by OTC drugs or prescription NSAIDs may respond well to weak opioids, the second step on the WHO ladder. These include hydrocodone and codeine, which is often mixed with a non-opioid pain reliever (Fiorinal, Phenaphen, or Tylenol with codeine).

Severe pain takes you another step up the ladder to strong opioids, most commonly morphine. Other strong opioids that are often prescribed include fentanyl, hydromorphone, levorphanol, methadone, and oxycodone. Opioids come in sustained-release forms for long-lasting relief as well as immediate-release forms that give faster but shorter-term relief and serve as "rescue medications" for breakthrough pain. Your doctor can continually raise the amount of opioid as needed to quell your pain, but the dose will be limited by common side effects such as constipation, nausea and vomiting, sleepiness, and slowed breathing.

Adjuvant drugs. Medications designed to treat other conditions may also relieve cancer pain, and are often used along with both non-opioids and opioids. Antidepressants (such as amitriptyline, nortriptyline, and desipramine) and anticonvulsants (carbamazepine, clonazepam, gabapentin, and phenytoin) can help control tingling or burning pain from nerve damage, while antihistamines (hydroxyzine and diphenhydramine) can ease nausea. Corticosteroids (dexamethasone and prednisone) may help relieve bone pain and inflammation—and often help stimulate a poor appetite.

Possible procedures. Sometimes cancer pain remains unrelieved even at the top rung of WHO's ladder. In such cases, other medical therapies and procedures may be used—including:

➤ **Nerve blocks** to prevent pain signals from registering in the brain

➤ **Injection therapies** that employ patient-controlled pumps that send painkiller into your system as needed

➤ **Neurosurgery or neuroablation,** in which nerves carrying pain signals are cut or destroyed

COMPLEMENTARY OPTIONS

Mainstream medicine is the mainstay of pain relief for cancer, but many major cancer centers offer clinics and integrative can-

CONTROLLING CANCER

Doctors call them risk factors, but they can just as easily be seen as control factors—behaviors that, if you take charge of them, may improve your odds of recovering from cancer or fending it off to begin with. While heredity plays a role in cancer development, most cases are connected with lifestyle choices. The prime example is smoking or regular exposure to secondhand smoke, which causes a third of all U.S. cancer deaths (and 85 percent of lung cancer deaths) each year, according to the National Cancer Institute. Smoking also increases the risk of cancers of the mouth, larynx, esophagus, pancreas, bladder, kidney, stomach, liver, prostate, colon, and rectum. Other potentially risk-raising lifestyle factors include a high-fat diet (linked with colon, uterine, and prostate cancers), exposure to sunlight (skin cancer), and excessive alcohol use (liver, mouth, throat, esophagus, and larynx cancers).

American Cancer Society
1599 Clifton Rd. N.E.
Atlanta, GA 30329
Phone: 800-227-2345
Website: www.cancer.org

Memorial Sloan-Kettering Cancer Center
1275 York Ave.
New York, NY 10021
Phone: 212-639-2000
Website: www.mskcc.org

National Cancer Institute
NCI Public Inquiries Office
Suite 3036A
6116 Executive Blvd.,
MSC8322
Bethesda, MD 20892-8322
Phone: 800-422-6237
Website: www.cancer.gov

University of Texas M.D. Anderson Cancer Center
1515 Holcombe Blvd.
Houston, TX 77030
Phone: 800-392-1611
Website: www.mdanderson.org

cer programs that incorporate both complementary and conventional treatments. It's estimated that about half of cancer patients have tried an unconventional method—which suggests that significant numbers of patients might benefit from non-drug therapies they haven't yet tried.

Mind/body methods. The full range of thought therapies described in chapter 3 are routinely prescribed for patients wrestling with cancer pain—including, for example, relaxation therapy, breathing exercises, and imagery. (*See "Parsing Pain from Within," below, for an exercise that combines all three.*) Research suggests that hypnosis may be particularly useful for managing cancer-related pain, according to the federal Agency for Healthcare Research and Quality.

Other non-drug therapies. A range of non-medical treatments may help relieve cancer pain. Among the most promising:

➤ **Acupuncture** appears to ease the nausea caused by chemotherapy drugs, and some evidence suggests that it may reduce the need for pain medication.

➤ **Transcutaneous electrical nerve stimulation (TENS)** may offer substantial relief from a particular pain, though results often last only while the electrical device is activated.

➤ **Touch therapies** such as massage and reflexology may help ease muscle tension, provide the soothing comfort of another person's touch, distract the mind from pain, and relieve anxiety that often accompanies serious illness.

PARSING PAIN FROM WITHIN

In a technique recommended by the National Cancer Institute, you use the teamed-up power of deep breathing and imagery in a meditative exercise that may help dissipate pain.

① Close your eyes and begin taking deep, slow, regular breaths. Count slowly to yourself as you breathe in, and again as you breathe out.

② As you breathe in and out, picture a ball of healing energy

forming deep within your chest or lungs. It may be helpful to imagine it as a white light.

③ While breathing in, imagine the air blowing the ball of energy to the area of your pain, where it heals and relaxes you.

④ While you breathe out, picture the ball blowing out of your body, taking your pain with it.

⑤ Continue picturing the energy ball healing and removing pain with each breath.

Many people find it surprising that small, repetitive movements like those required for typing, sewing, computing, or playing the piano can wreak havoc on the wrist. A more pleasant surprise is this: The pain of carpal tunnel syndrome (CTS) doesn't have to make you give up your daily activities or favorite pastimes—as long as you pace yourself and follow some simple steps. Your goal is to keep muscles, tendons, and nerves in the hands and wrist supple, strong, and resilient, and to treat remaining pain directly.

Understanding the Pain

The carpal tunnel is just what it sounds like: a narrow passageway. But in this case, it's a passageway made of ligament and bone that burrows through the center of the wrist. The median nerve, which supplies both sensation and movement to the thumb, index finger, long finger, and ring finger, runs through this tunnel—along with tendons that allow the hand to close. Steady and repetitive hand movements (grasping, twisting, and turning), especially when they involve vibrations (as when using computer keyboards, hammers, power tools, or certain musical instruments), can cause the tendons to swell, narrowing the tunnel and pinching the median nerve. What can result are the hallmarks of CTS, which include:

➤ Pain, tingling, or numbness in the fingers and hand
➤ Shooting pains through the wrist and forearm
➤ Difficulty clenching the fist or grasping small objects

SELF-CARE STRATEGIES

Rest. Overcoming CTS generally begins with an ending—of the repetitive movement that caused the pain. If that's not possible, you should at least alter your pattern of movement. Give your hands frequent breaks from activity, flexing fingers and

INSTANT ACTION

■ Stop any and all repetitive hand movements, like typing, playing the piano, etc.

■ Take a standard dose of an anti-inflammatory painkiller like ibuprofen.

■ If pain is intense, apply ice packs to the wrist to reduce swelling.

■ If pain is subtle and numbing, apply heat to the hand or wrist to increase blood circulation and reduce pain.

■ Put on a brace or splint to prevent further pain-inducing movements.

■ If you can't halt pain-producing movement altogether, take more frequent breaks to give tendons a chance to rest and recover.

CARPAL TUNNEL SYNDROME
Ailments

shaking hands at least once an hour. Try to make tendons and muscles move in new ways that don't cause pain with simple stretches and exercises of the wrist and fingers.

Exercise. Gentle exercises can go a long way toward relieving pain and improving function in carpel tunnel syndrome. The most effective exercises may be as simple as:

➤ Rotating your hands in a circle from the wrist, first in one direction, then another

➤ Wrapping your fingers in a rubber band and spreading them apart

➤ Squeezing and manipulating a wad of clay or Silly Putty

Improved positioning. You may want to consult a physical or occupational therapist for pointers on how to modify your movements, but simple changes you can make on your own can help keep pain at bay. In particular, adjust your posture while working at a desk to keep your hands and wrists stable and properly positioned. Sit upright with your spine against the back of your chair and your feet flat on the floor. Wrists should be straight, not flexed up or down, but your shoulders and arms should be relaxed, with your elbows at your sides. Keep the screen at eye level and avoid slouching over your work.

Splint or brace. A physical therapist may recommend using a splint or brace to keep the wrist from bending so there's less pressure on the nerve. (Most patients reserve this treatment for nighttime, but a splint may be worn around the clock for severe symptoms.)

Ice. When pain is especially intense, apply ice for 10 to 15 minutes every hour or so while awake to constrict blood vessels and reduce swelling.

Heat. Just turning up the thermostat in your house and making the room warmer can help ease pain

Ergonomic tools. Check out websites such as www.wrist-paincentral.com or www.ctsplace.com for information and products such as wearable supports and wraps that can help shore up the wrist, or ergonomic devices that support the wrist or arm while you work at a computer. Just keep in mind that information from a website shouldn't take the place of medical advice from your physician. Talk to your doctor for guidance on the products that may be most appropriate for you.

Fist exercises. Simply making a fist three different ways can help relieve pain by exercising tendons in the hand, according to the American Physical Therapy Association. Here's what the APTA recommends:

1. Start with your fingers in a straight position.

2. Curl your fingers at the middle joint so they make a hook, with fingertips pressed against the top of your palm. Hold for five seconds, then relax. Repeat four times.

3. From the starting position, make a straight fist with fingers pressed flat against your palm. Hold five seconds, relax, and repeat four times.

4. From the starting position, make a full fist, hold five seconds, relax, and repeat four times.

Stop smoking. Tobacco can make CTS worse by hindering the nourishing flow of blood to small vessels in the hand.

MEDICAL MEASURES

Medications. CTS treatment usually starts with a non-steroidal anti-inflammatory (NSAID) such as ibuprofen (Advil, Motrin, and Nuprin) or naproxen (Aleve), available over the counter. If this doesn't reduce pain and swelling, a doctor may prescribe a stronger anti-inflammatory medication or a corticosteroid such as cortisone. Corticosteroids are usually injected into the wrist, but a new technique called iontophresis uses an electric current to send molecules of the drug through the skin and into the carpal tunnel. It's less painful than a shot, but may also be less effective.

Surgery. If less conservative approaches fail, and CTS symptoms continue persistently or intermittently for a year or more, a form of surgery called carpal tunnel release may be needed to take pressure off the compressed median nerve. The most common procedure involves cutting the transverse carpal ligament, a tough band of tissue that forms one side of the carpal tunnel. When the operation is done using endoscopy, tiny incisions allow doctors to perform the operation using a telescopic device with a tiny TV camera that allows the doctor to see and work inside the carpal tunnel.

Physical therapy. Treatments may include ultrasound, diathermy (deep heat therapy), transcutaneous electrical nerve

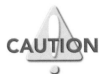

CAUTION

Be wary of supplements purporting that vitamin B_6 relieves carpal tunnel syndrome. This 30-year-old claim is not borne out by scientific studies, according to the National Institutes of Health. In fact, excessive doses of vitamin B_6 may actually cause nerve damage. The National Academy of Sciences' Institute of Medicine has established 100 milligrams as a tolerable daily limit, though B_6 proponents generally suggest daily doses ranging up to 200 mg. There's no need for pills: A varied diet including B_6-rich foods such as beef, bananas, fish, and rice will provide all of the vitamin that you need.

CARPAL TUNNEL SYNDROME

Ailments

SEX AND CTS

Women are about three times more likely than men to develop carpal tunnel syndrome, for several possible reasons:

■ Women's generally smaller wrists are more vulnerable because the carpal tunnel is narrower.

■ Women hold more jobs or engage in more hobbies with repetitive hand movements.

■ Hormonal changes due to the menstrual cycle, pregnancy, and menopause may increase risk.

But plenty of men get CTS as well, and the sexes share a number of risk factors, including health conditions such as thyroid problems, diabetes, obesity, and rheumatoid arthritis. Participation in wrist-stressing sports such as golf, tennis, archery, competitive shooting, and rock climbing can also bring on CTS.

stimulation (TENS), hydrotherapy, and alternating hot and cold packs. A physical therapist will also teach you exercises to prevent further injury..

COMPLEMENTARY OPTIONS

Acupuncture. A consensus panel of the National Institutes of Health reports that acupuncture, when used in conjunction with medical treatment, may help relieve the pain of carpal tunnel syndrome.

Yoga. By stretching and strengthening joints in the upper body, yoga can also help treat carpal tunnel syndrome. According to a small study in *The Journal of the American Medical Association,* CTS patients who preformed yoga had fewer symptoms than those who relied on wrist splints or used no treatment at all.

Chiropractic. Practitioners help CTS patients by manipulating misaligned or fixated joints to relieve pressure on the median nerve. Adjustments are made not only to the wrist but also to other areas affected by the median nerve—the arm, shoulder, and neck.

In the late 1930s, a neurologist's report in a British medical journal discussed a "pain worse than pain"— a previously known but little-understood agony now called central pain syndrome. Central pain is the frontier of pain medicine: Caused by damage to the central nervous system, often within the brain itself, it's maddeningly resistant to self-care—and medical treatments for it are less effective than for other types of pain. But it's important not to give up hope. "Central pain is difficult to treat—but not impossible," says Michael R. Clark, M.D., director of the chronic pain treatment program at Johns Hopkins University's department of psychiatry and behavioral medicine. "The single biggest problem is that patients—and their doctors— get into a rut where they assume nothing more can be done. But there's always a next step."

Understanding the Pain

Central pain syndrome has other names as well—thalamic-pain syndrome, Dejerine-Roussy syndrome, posterior thalamic syndrome, retrolenticular syndrome, and central poststroke syndrome—due to its having a variety of potential causes. These include brain or spinal cord injury and stroke, along with systemic diseases such as multiple sclerosis (MS) and acquired immunodeficiency syndrome (AIDS). The source of pain appears to be associated with lesions on the spinal cord, lower brainstem, or, especially, the thalamus, a part of the brain responsible for sensing pain.

An estimated 100,000 Americans suffer from central pain syndrome, which causes a constant burning, aching, or cutting pain, perhaps affecting one half of the body, at least one limb, or the face. Often, pain centers in the chest, feet, or hands. Electrical sensations of cold, tingling, or exposed nerves may mix in with deep, steady pain, and affected areas can be extremely sensitive to temperature or touch, particularly sensations of cold—or even the light pressure of clothing.

CENTRAL PAIN SYNDROME
Ailments

SELF-CARE STRATEGIES

Expert help. If rank-and-file doctors often throw up their hands when treating pain from other conditions, they're even more likely with central pain to decide there's nothing more they can do. But that's simply wrong, says Clark. "I get patients at the end of their rope who say, 'My doctor gave me three different drugs in three years; what else can I try?' And I say, 'About 50 others.'" Your primary-care physician may not understand all the options available. If you feel you've reached the limits of your doctor's knowledge or ability, consult a neurologist or pain specialist—experts more likely to understand the nature of central pain and have experience dealing with it.

Forward focus. "You should never get to a point where you say, 'This is my last hope,'" says Clark. "There's always something else you can try." If what your doctor prescribes doesn't bring adequate relief, press him or her for more options. Go through treatments systematically, always asking what should follow. "You'll make progress with experience, practice, education—and a willingness to take the next step," says Clark.

Realistic goals. At the same time, it's important to understand that treatment may not make pain go away entirely. Keeping your assumptions grounded can guard against disappointment and the pain-magnifying depression that can sometimes result. That's not a concession to futility: Look for treatment to provide a measure of relief by at least taking the edge off pain.

MEDICAL MEASURES

Adjuvants first. The first-line medical defense usually rests on antidepressants and anticonvulsants, depending on what's behind the condition. People with central pain following stroke, for example, appear to do better with tricyclic antidepressants such as amitriptyline or nortriptyline than people with spinal cord injury or multiple sclerosis. On the other hand, MS patients tend to respond better to anticonvulsants such as gabapentin, carbamazepine, or clonazepam. Generally, experts suggest slowly working up to as high a dose as necessary and tolerable to see if the drugs will help.

Opioids. How well opioid painkillers such as morphine

subdue central pain is a matter of debate: Some doctors say they help only a little or not at all, while other physicians claim better results. Most agree, however, that opioids help less against central pain than other types of pain. Still, with all the drugs available, "your options are virtually unlimited," says Clark. "Failure is never failure—it's just more information about what does or doesn't work." An unmistakable benefit of some opioids, for example, is sedation to keep the nervous system as quiet and stress-free as possible.

More medication methods. A number of other drugs can be tried as well, including the blood pressure drugs clonidine and propranolol, which have been shown to block the release of pain-related chemical messengers in the nervous system. On the lookout for alternatives, doctors sometimes try combinations of drugs. For example, in one small study, half of patients with central pain obtained long-lasting relief with doxepin, an antidepressant, teamed with propranolol. Another alternative for some patients is intravenous treatment with lidocaine, a short-acting local anesthetic, which—though its effects on central pain haven't been carefully studied in controlled trials—also appears to be of some limited benefit.

Nerve-numbing options. In some cases, neurosurgeons are called in for operations on the spinal cord that may help relieve pain by disrupting nerve connections that send signals to the brain. One of the most promising of these procedures, called the DREZ (dorsal root entry zone) lesion, has had a success rate of about 50 percent—though even when it's successful, it may not provide long-term relief.

COMPLEMENTARY OPTIONS

A far less invasive alternative to surgery is using transcutaneous electrical nerve stimulation (TENS), in which electrodes worn on the skin send small amounts of electricity into the body. In one study, 7 out of 11 people with central pain from spinal cord injury responded well to TENS. If that doesn't work, it's possible to try a more involved—and still-experimental—technique called deep brain stimulation, in which implanted electrodes deliver electrical impulses to the brain.

Ailments

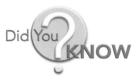

There was a time when few doctors took chronic fatigue syndrome (CFS) seriously: Because physical exams didn't suggest an explanation for patients' complaints of overwhelming fatigue and nearly constant pain, the problem was dismissed as largely psychological. Today, however, researchers recognize CFS as a real illness—one that demands real treatment. Thanks to a greater understanding of energy-conserving lifestyle changes and fatigue-fighting medications, it's possible to overcome CFS.

Understanding the Pain

If you have CFS, you're not just tired all the time (a common complaint even among healthy adults)—you're also plagued by flu-like symptoms, including joint and muscle pain, sore throat, and headache. But unlike the flu, chronic fatigue syndrome lingers for months, even years, often making it difficult to go about daily business or socialize with family and friends.

Despite progress in understanding, CFS still baffles researchers, who have yet to uncover its exact cause or cure. Its myriad symptoms, which vary from patient to patient, long defied simple definition, but in 1994 researchers concluded that a diagnosis rests on two main criteria:

➤ Severe chronic fatigue lasting at least six months and not caused by another known medical condition

➤ At least four other specific symptoms that persist or recur during that six-month period. These symptoms include problems with concentration or short-term memory, sore throat, tender lymph nodes, muscle pain, joint aches (but no swelling or redness), headache, unrefreshing sleep, and malaise that lasts more than 24 hours after exertion.

Between 20 and 50 percent of CFS patients also report a wide range of other complaints, including abdominal pain, chest pain, chronic cough, diarrhea, dizziness, dry eyes or mouth, ear-

INSTANT ACTION

■ Keep an energy diary, which allows you to pinpoint what activities or emotional upsets are most likely to trigger symptoms.

■ Become an efficiency expert: Plan your day around your highest peaks of energy. Strike unimportant tasks from your to-do list, or delegate them to someone else.

■ Power nap: Determine whether your lost energy is best restored with a single long nap, or shorter—but more frequent—periods of rest or relaxation.

aches, fever, irregular heartbeat, jaw pain, morning stiffness, nausea, night sweats, shortness of breath, or tingling sensations. But there's light at the end of the tunnel: Fatigue and pain (along with psychological difficulties that often go with them) are usually worst during the first year or two. After that, you have a 50/50 chance of full recovery within five years—and the vast majority of people with CFS eventually recover.

Combating Chronic Fatigue and Pain

If you have CFS, "moderation in all things" is not just a philosophy, it's a health plan. Most doctors advise patients to pace themselves and avoid emotional stress and physical exertion, which can trigger exhaustion and a relapse of symptoms. It's vital to eat frequently (for a steady supply of energy) but not overindulge, sleep enough but not too much, and exercise regularly to maintain physical condition but not to the point of fatigue. Meanwhile, symptoms can be managed to reduce pain and restore normal life as much as possible.

SELF-CARE STRATEGIES

Keep it moving. It may seem odd to exercise as a remedy for fatigue, but most doctors advise engaging in physical activity as much as you can manage—"daily if possible," says Timothy J. Craig, D.O., professor of medicine at Pennsylvania State University College of Medicine in Hershey. In one 12-week study in England, more than half of CFS patients who walked, swam, or cycled 5 to 30 minutes a day reported feeling much better. It's wise to lay off exercise when symptoms are most severe—but don't let yourself go too long: A lengthy hiatus decreases general physical fitness as well as mood, energy level, and mental functioning. Get back into action as soon as you can.

Eat a well-balanced diet. If you're prone to food sensitivities or intolerances—not unusual with CFS—resist the temptation to severely restrict your diet, which can deprive you of proper nutrition and undermine your recovery. Usually, eliminating just a few offending foods with the help of a doctor or nutritionist can improve symptoms such as

---

CHECKLIST FOR RELIEF

✔ Self-Care Strategies

Regular exercise	p. 71
Adequate rest	
Balanced diet	
Increased fiber intake	
Better sleep habits	p.141

✔ Medical Measures

NSAIDs	p. 41
Tricyclic antidepressants	p. 48
Selective serotonin reuptake inhibitors	
Anticonvulsants	p. 49

✔ Complementary Options

Cognitive behavioral therapy	
Meditation	p. /8
Yoga	p. 96
Hypnosis	p. 80
St. John's wort	p.127

BEYOND YUPPIES

During the 1980s, when there was a surge of scientific and lay interest in chronic fatigue syndrome, the condition seemed mostly to affect well-educated, affluent women in their 30s and 40s, leading to the nickname "yuppie flu"—a misnomer. Today, it's clear that susceptibility to CFS doesn't depend on age, educational background, or financial status, though it's still most common among women.

MAKING THE GRADE IN EXERCISE

Research suggests that a graded exercise program—working out at an increasingly intense level as your condition allows—can help CFS sufferers kick their symptoms. In a 2001 study, more than 80 percent of CFS patients who put themselves on a gradually intensifying plan reported improvement—and the benefits lasted for at least a year. To set up your own graded workout schedule, experts advise you:

■ Start with just 3 to 5 minutes of moderate exercise every day.

■ Increase your activity by 20 percent every two to three weeks, if you are able.

■ Don't work out beyond your established limit to keep from overexerting yourself.

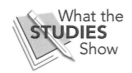

What the STUDIES Show

Doctors tend to report that people with CFS have normal physical exams, but a new study suggests otherwise: Kids with CFS are three and a half times more likely to have hyperflexible joints than healthy children, say researchers at Johns Hopkins Children's Center. The ability to bend fingers backward or hyperextend elbows and knees likely doesn't in itself cause CFS, but the link may lead to more insight into how symptoms develop.

headache, muscle pain, and malaise. At the same time, adding rich sources of fiber, such as fruits and vegetables with peels, may help relieve constipation, another common symptom. "Frequently, irritable bowel syndrome occurs with CFS, and adding roughage helps reduce bowel pain," says Craig.

Practical help. One reason CFS patients feel so exhausted is lack of quality sleep. Try to control your sleep environment. If light filters through your windows at night, get thicker, room-darkening shades. If you have trouble getting comfortable in bed, invest in a new mattress or pillow. If noise disturbs you, try a white noise machine or one that plays ocean sounds.

MEDICAL MEASURES

Common pain relievers. For mild muscle and joint pain, headache, and fever, over-the-counter nonsteroidal anti-inflammatory drugs (NSAIDs) such as aspirin, ibuprofen (Advil, Motrin, Nuprin), and naproxen (Aleve) will usually provide adequate relief. For persistent pain, your doctor may want to prescribe newer COX-2 inhibitor NSAIDs such as celecoxib (Celebrex).

Tricyclic antidepressants. If NSAIDs don't do the trick, a tricyclic agent may be worth a try. Although classified as antidepressants, tricyclic agents also appear to promote better-quality sleep and reduce generalized pain, making them particularly beneficial for CFS. Options include doxepin (Adapin and Sinequan), amitriptyline (Elavil, Etrafon, Limbitrol, and Triavil), desipramine (Norpramin), and nortriptyline (Pamelor). Selective serotonin reuptake inhibitors (such as Prozac and Wellbutrin), another type of antidepressant, may be prescribed, though research hasn't revealed particularly notable benefits for CFS.

Anti-seizure medications. Many people with CFS also take clonazepam (Klonopin), an anticonvulsant that controls insomnia and, some patients say, clears mental fogginess and relieves flu-like achiness.

Whenever using drugs normally taken for psychological problems, your doctor will typically start you with a lower-than-usual dose, because regular therapeutic doses of these medications tend to increase fatigue in CFS patients.

COMPLEMENTARY OPTIONS

Psychological therapy. CFS takes a toll mentally and physically, and cognitive behavioral therapy, in which you learn to challenge unhealthy negative thinking, can prove helpful for calming both mind and body. Studies show that cognitive-behavioral therapy helps people with CFS develop better coping skills, relieving hopelessness and distress often felt when facing an uncertain future of pain and exhaustion. In one study, patients who received cognitive therapy along with standard medical care spent more time up and functioning than did those using standard treatments alone.

Relaxation methods. Meditation, yoga, and hypnosis have all been reported to help relieve the malaise of CFS, though their benefits have not been closely studied.

Helpful herbs. Although many herbs are purported to help CFS, few seem to be effective. One worth considering, however, is St. John's wort, best known as a treatment for mild depression. In one study, St. John's wort seemed to decrease fatigue in people with CFS, regardless of whether they also reported depression as a symptom.

READY RESOURCES

Centers for Disease Control and Prevention
National Center for Infectious Diseases
Division of Viral and Rickettsial Diseases
Atlanta, GA 30333
Phone: 888-232-3228
Website:
www.cdc.gov/ncidod/dvrd

CFIDS Association of America
P.O. Box 220398
Charlotte, NC 28222-0398
Phone: 800-442-3437
Fax: 704-365-9755
Website: www.cfids.org

National Chronic Fatigue Syndrome and Fibromyalgia Association
P.O. Box 18426
Kansas City, MO 64133
Phone: 816-313-2000
Fax: 816-524-6782
Website: www.ncfsfa.org

ON THE HORIZON

Ongoing research into the best treatments for CFS reveals some promising results with:

■ **Ampligen,** a drug that uses the body's genetic material (DNA and RNA) to reprogram diseased cells to fight illness. In clinical trials, patients have reported improvement, even full recovery, in mental and physical function.

■ **Corticosteroids,** which reduce inflammation. Researchers report that low-dose hydrocortisone improved fatigue and disability among CFS patients in one study. However, side effects may present a problem.

■ **NADH,** a form of the coenzyme nicotinamide adenine dinucleotide. This nutritional supplement may alleviate exhaustion and improve cognitive function in CFS patients, say investigators.

During the Civil War, a doctor named Silas Weir Mitchell reported that some injured veterans complained of burning pain that persisted and spread long after their wounds had healed. He dubbed the disorder "causalgia," which means "hot pain," and concluded it was linked to nerve damage. Modern doctors, who still don't know what causes the condition, call it complex regional pain syndrome. If the battle with CRPS begins within a few months of onset, patients can recover from the disorder completely.

Understanding the Pain

Pain from CRPS seems wildly out of proportion to the injuries that appear to set it off—sprains, fractures, traumas from car accidents, surgical incisions, and even bug bites. Many patients can't pinpoint a trigger. Whatever the cause, pain from the injury fails to completely clear up. Instead, burning, aching, or searing pain develops and gets worse over time—sometimes kicking in weeks after the original injury heals. Pain often occurs on a limb, but sometimes hits the face or trunk, and—if untreated—tends to progressively creep over the entire area, affecting skin, bone, muscle, and joints.

Doctors identify two types of complex regional pain syndrome. The most common, CRPS I (sometimes called reflex sympathetic dystrophy) doesn't involve nerve injury, but—as Silas Weir Mitchell surmised—CRPS II does. But both types share basic symptoms, which generally progress through three stages:

Stage 1: Burning pain occurs at the injury site, perhaps with muscle spasms and stiff joints. The slightest sensation—light touch, contact with clothing—causes pain, a condition known as allodynia. Skin in the painful area may look blotchy and be warm to the touch, while hair there grows rapidly. Timetable: one to three months.

Stage 2: Pain gets worse, swelling spreads, hair and nail growth slows, and skin becomes bluish, sweaty, and cool. To

INSTANT ACTION

■ Apply a hot water bottle or heating pad to the affected area.

■ Take deep, calming breaths to make pain seem less daunting.

■ Tame pain-magnifying stress by using your inner voice to reassure yourself: "I can handle pain—I've done it before."

contain the pain, the patient may keep the limb still, making it stiffen from disuse. As a result, muscles can weaken and bones may lose density. Timetable: three to six months or longer.

Stage 3: Constant pain now involves the entire limb, perhaps spreading to the opposite one. Muscles atrophy, severely limiting movement, and changes to skin and bones may become irreversible. Timetable: more than six months.

SELF-CARE STRATEGIES

Heat and cold. While a physical therapist will make temperature treatments part of your scheduled sessions, you can also treat yourself at home. Ask your therapist for advice on what's appropriate, but you'll likely benefit from soothing hot baths, hot pads, and maybe hot-and-cold contrast baths.

Stress management. It's important to fight CRPS's mental and emotional wounds, which can sear your spirit along with your body, potentially making pain worse. Staying physically active is one of the best ways to tame the tension of CRPS; it calms your mind and can help you physically relieve pain. Even when you're sitting still, you can practice deep breathing and stress inoculation, in which you speak to yourself using calming statements such as "Pain won't get the best of me."

Emotional control. Depression and anxiety are cousins to stress, and should be tackled because they not only make you miserable but can make pain worse. Physical activity helps here too. Cognitive behavioral therapy can help you use affirming statements to turn aside gloomy feelings.

MEDICAL MEASURES

Physical therapy. The main goal of CRPS treatment is to keep your body from becoming weaker and less mobile due to inactivity that—ironically—actually makes pain worse. Physical therapy is the treatment that clinical studies show most clearly to be of benefit. Persistence pays off, but it is hard to accomplish because the pain becomes greater before it begins to subside. Many patients give up too soon. To combat the hypersensitivity of allodynia, therapists use a critical touch therapy in which your practitioner gently runs over skin with very soft, light materials, working up to heavier, rougher textures to gradually build toler-

CHECKLIST FOR RELIEF

✔ **Self-Care Strategies**

Heat and cold	p. 88
Deep breathing	p. 71
Stress inoculation	p. 72
Cognitive behavioral therapy	

✔ **Medical Measures**

Touch therapy	
Exercise therapy	p. 71
Nerve blocks	p. 55
Antidepressants	p.136
Anticonvulsants	p. 49
Sympathectomy	
Spinal cord stimulation	

✔ **Complementary Options**

TENS	p.102
Biofeedback	p. 79
Acupuncture	p.113

American RSD Hope Group
P.O. Box 875
Harrison, ME 04040-0875
Phone: 207-583-4589
Website: www.rsdhope.org

Reflex Sympathetic Dystrophy Syndrome Association of America (RSDSA)
P.O. Box 502
Milford, CT 06460
Phone: 203-877-3790
Fax: 203-882-8362
Website: www.rsds.org

ance to sensation. Once you're comfortable enough, light exercises to promote flexibility and strength can be introduced. As you improve, you'll be able to move on to more intense motion exercises, strength training (perhaps using weights), and aerobic conditioning—all of which can help relieve pain over time.

Nerve blocks. Studies suggest that most people with CRPS can benefit from nerve blocks, which numb nerves with an injected anesthetic such as lidocaine. Nerve blocks can also make early physical therapy sessions tolerable for patients.

Oral medications. Antidepressants such as amitriptyline, nortriptyline, and doxepin seem to help CRPS patients both by reducing pain and easing the pain-promoting effects of depression. Bonus: Because they're sedating, patients otherwise kept awake by pain often sleep better. The anticonvulsant gabapentin also seems to have analgesic effects for CRPS, although it tends to be most effective when used with other pain relievers. Experts differ on the usefulness of opioids. Corticosteroids may help patients whose original injury caused inflammation.

Surgical options. If you're disabled by CRPS and nerve blocks provide only brief relief, your doctor might suggest a sympathectomy—surgery that kills the sympathetic nerves that lead to the painful area. Be cautious about this solution: Pain sometimes returns after six months, and there's a risk of developing a new type of pain known as post-sympathectomy syndrome. If all else fails, a pain specialist might recommend spinal cord stimulation, also known as dorsal column stimulation, in which an electrode inside the spine provides low-voltage electrical impulses that distract the brain from feeling pain.

COMPLEMENTARY OPTIONS

TENS. Some doctors recommend trying transcutaneous electrical nerve stimulation, which uses a special device to apply brief pulses of electrical energy to painful areas.

Biofeedback. Some doctors suggest that the control patients feel with biofeedback can both help relieve pain and ease anxiety that can make pain more intense.

Acupuncture. Though not well studied for CRPS, acupuncture may help relieve discomfort by stimulating points associated with the area that hurts.

I t's not a social disease, but if you have endometriosis, some of your 10 closest female friends probably do too: It's among the most common gynecological disorders, affecting up to 20 percent of American women of childbearing age. Compare notes and you'll find that symptoms can vary enormously: Some women have little or no pain at all, while others suffer from cramps, aching, or other pain all month long. But an end to pain is always in sight. Symptoms quit when menstruation does—either because of menopause or pregnancy. Best of all, there's no reason to suffer until symptoms go into natural remission. You can usually manage endometriosis pain with lifestyle changes and medical therapies.

Understanding the Pain

"Endometriosis" refers to the endometrium—the lining of the uterus. Each month, the endometrium builds up and is flushed out during menstruation. Sometimes, however, microscopic bits of uterine tissue go AWOL, breaking away from the lining and embedding themselves elsewhere in the body, often in the pelvic area. These transplanted growths may continue to follow the menstrual cycle, thickening and then breaking down in response to hormonal fluctuations—without being flushed from the body. Stuck in unnatural locations such as the ovaries or bladder, growths cause swelling and inflammation, and over time develop into cysts, scars, and adhesions. That often leads to pain such as:

➤ Heavy aching in the lower abdomen, back, and rectum that may radiate into the vagina and upper legs

➤ Cramps that may begin a week or two before menstruation starts

➤ Increasingly uncomfortable periods

During your period, you may find it hurts to move your bowels or urinate, and pain may occur during and after sexual inter-

INSTANT ACTION

- Soak in a tub of warm water.

- Add a few drops of soothing juniper, peppermint, or marjoram oils to warm water in a sitz bath or tub.

- If heat doesn't help, apply a cold pack.

- Combine therapies with contrast baths.

- Take an NSAID or acetaminophen.

- Drink water or juice instead of coffee, tea, and colas to reduce pain and improve bladder and bowel function.

ENDOMETRIOSIS

Ailments

course at any time of the month—the reason many women finally seek help. Severe scarring and organ damage may affect fertility, making endometriosis a top cause of female infertility, according to the National Institute of Child Health & Human Reproduction. "Up to 30 percent of women with difficulty conceiving have endometriosis confirmed," says Magdy Milad, M.D., associate professor of obstetrics and gynecology at Northwestern University's Feinberg School of Medicine.

SELF-CARE STRATEGIES

Heat or cold. Most people find that applying heat to the lower abdomen with a hot-water bottle or heating pad helps relieve cramps and soothe aching muscles. But if that doesn't work, try cold treatment, which feels better to some women. The best bet for convenience and comfort is a flexible, frozen gel pack (sold in most pharmacies), but if you don't have one handy, put ice cubes in a plastic bag and wrap it in a cloth—or, for added pliability, freeze a wet cloth in a plastic bag and wrap the bag in a second cloth.

Contrast sitz baths. To help ease pelvic inflammation with a hot-and-cold combination, sit in a sitz bath (a toilet-fitting basin available at medical supply stores or some pharmacies) filled with hot water for three minutes, then switch to a second sitz bath filled with ice water for one minute. Go back and forth three more times, twice a day. Repeat the process three or four times a week except during menstruation. For added pain relief, try adding a few aromatic drops of juniper, peppermint, or marjoram oils—thought to ease endometriosis pain—to a warm-water sitz bath or tub.

Kegel exercises. You'll feel less pain if you strengthen pelvic and pubic muscles, which eases bladder problems (such as frequent urination). Bonus: The exercises also make sexual intercourse more pleasurable. The best way to power up your pelvis is to do Kegel exercises at least three times a day, in the morning, afternoon, and at night—and whenever else you can manage. To perform them, tighten and hold the muscles that start and stop urine flow for a count of 10, then release them for a count of 10. Repeat 10 to 15 times.

Cutting caffeine. Some experts suggest you can gain significant relief by cutting back on caffeine, which appears to make pain worse in some women. Drinking water or juice instead not only replaces caffeine, it improves bladder and bowel function, which can also help ease pain from endometriosis.

Oily fish. Sardines, mackerel, and other oily fish contain omega-3 fatty acids, natural "good" fats that are thought to have anti-inflammatory qualities. If adding these foods to your diet doesn't seem to make a difference, consider taking a supplement, with your doctor's approval.

Fiber. Dietary fiber from food such as lentils and whole-grain breads may help reduce pain by preventing constipation, which tends to make symptoms of endometriosis worse.

Sanitary napkins. Some women find they experience more cramping when using tampons, leading doctors to sometimes recommend sanitary napkins instead.

MEDICAL MEASURES

Oral pain relievers. Mild to moderate endometriosis pain often responds to over-the-counter nonsteroidal anti-inflammatory drugs (NSAIDs) such as ibuprofen and naproxen. To avoid gastrointestinal problems common with regular use of standard NSAIDs, some women gain similar relief with fewer side effects by using acetaminophen (Tylenol) or prescription COX-2 inhibitor NSAIDs (Celebrex, Vioxx, and Bextra).

Hormonal treatment. Fooling the body into thinking you've hit menopause or you're pregnant suspends the monthly stimulation of hormones, making endometrial growths shrink and disappear—along with the pain they bring. These therapies, which bring pain relief to about 80 percent of endometriosis sufferers, include:

➤ A new class of drugs called gonadotropin-releasing hormone (GnRH) agonists. These block luteinizing hormone and follicle-stimulating hormone, which induce ovulation and menstruation. Examples include Synarel (a nasal spray), Lupron (a shot), and Zoladex (implants). Though effective, their side effects—including menopausal symptoms such as hot flashes, vaginal dryness, mood changes, and an increased risk of osteoporosis—limit use to six months.

➤ Taking oral contraceptives (such as Lo/Ovral and Ortho-

Novum) all month long, rather than just three weeks of the cycle. This creates a "pseudopregnancy" state that prevents ovulation. Your doctor will advise you on how long to use birth control pills containing estrogen and progesterone, which can generally be used for nine months or longer, but may produce side effects such as weight gain and spotting.

➤ Oral or injectable progestin-only therapy. Natural progesterone (prometrium) or synthetic versions (such as Provera, Depo-Provera, and Norethindrone) continuously suppress ovulation and endometriosis growth, and can be used for months or years. Side effects are similar to oral contraceptives—but they also pose a rare risk of bone loss. Long-term use has become controversial and probably has substantial risks.

➤ A weak synthetic version of the male hormone testosterone, called danazol (Danocrine). Danazol creates an artificial menopause by preventing the surge of luteinizing hormone and follicle-stimulating hormone. Treatment usually lasts just three to six months because of the risk of unpleasant side effects such as weight gain, bloating, and high cholesterol, increased body hair growth, and deepening of the voice—reasons this therapy is less common than other treatments, says Milad.

Surgical solutions. "If a woman has pain that interferes with daily functioning despite taking hormonal therapy, she should consider surgery," says Milad. The least invasive procedure, laparoscopy, uses a lighted tube to see inside the abdomen through a tiny incision and remove damaged tissue. Larger growths or affected organs may require a full incision, known as laparotomy. Both procedures spare healthy surrounding tissue, allowing patients to continue bearing children. However, severe cases with lots of scarring may require hysterectomy, or removal of the uterus (sometimes along with the ovaries and fallopian tubes), making pregnancy impossible.

WONDERING ABOUT WANDERING TISSUE

Why does endometrial tissue wander and settle into places it doesn't belong? No one knows for sure, but some researchers believe that during menstruation, some of the tissue backs up through the fallopian tubes and implants in the pelvis or abdominal cavity. Others suspect that some women are more susceptible to endometriosis due to a faulty immune system, which fails to destroy displaced cells. Still others theorize that a genetic component leaves certain families particularly vulnerable to the condition, and family history certainly is a risk factor: A woman whose mother or sister has endometriosis is at six times the risk of the general population.

COMPLEMENTARY OPTIONS

Acupressure. Applying pressure at an acupoint on the ankle (also used for acupuncture) associated with urinary and genital problems seems to control endometriosis symptoms for some women. See an acupuncturist for an initial treatment, and ask if you can use the technique—which involves stimulating the point by strapping a rubber device around the ankle—at home.

Hormone-helping herbs. Some practitioners recommend using chaste tree or dong quai, herbs believed to promote normal balances of estrogen and progesterone during menstruation. Red raspberry leaf and valerian, herbal remedies suggested to reduce menstrual pain, may also benefit endometriosis. Be sure to check with your doctor before adding herbs to your pain management program, particularly if you are (or plan to be) pregnant or nursing.

Anti-inflammatory spices. Both ginger and turmeric are thought to have anti-inflammatory properties that may help relieve pain from endometriosis, although no conclusive studies have been conducted to confirm these benefits.

Gamma-linolenic acid (GLA). This omega-6 fatty acid—another of the body's "good" fats—is thought to relieve conditions that involve inflammation. Though little research has been done, GLA (found in evening primrose oil) has been suggested to relieve pain and other symptoms of endometriosis in part because there's evidence it helps with premenstrual syndrome.

Relaxation techniques. To help you cope with pain and stress associated with endometriosis, you may find it helpful to practice methods such as meditation, deep breathing, imagery, and yoga.

READY RESOURCES

Endometriosis Association
International Headquarters
8585 N. 76th Place
Milwaukee, WI 53223
Phone: 414-355-2000/800-992-3636
Fax: 414-355-6065
Website: www.endometriosisassn.org

National Institute of Child Health and Human Development
Building 31, Room 2A32, MSC 2425
31 Center Dr.
Bethesda, MD 20892-2425
Phone: 800-370-2943
Website: www.nichd.nih.gov

Doctors can't pin the all-over achiness and constant fatigue of fibromyalgia on any known disease—nor can they explain other common symptoms of fibromyalgia, such as headaches or stomach problems. People who have fibromyalgia often fall into a cyclical pattern in which pain interferes with sleep, exhaustion aggravates pain, and pain causes more interrupted sleep. The cycle can be broken with self-help and medical measures that not only treat pain but shatter links in the chain of misery.

Understanding the Pain

Fibromyalgia affects an estimated 6 to 8 million Americans, mostly women. That makes fibromyalgia symptoms among the most common complaints brought to rheumatologists today, according to Gary S. Firestein, M.D., chief of the division of rheumatology, allergy, and immunology at the University of California-San Diego School of Medicine. Though blood tests and X rays generally reveal no abnormalities, fibromyalgia may be diagnosed if you've had pain in at least 11 of 18 specific "tender points" (knees, elbows, hip joints, shoulders, and neck, for example) for more than three months. Beyond pain (which can be aching, stabbing, or burning) and poor sleep, other symptoms may include:

➤ Numbness or tingling in hands and feet
➤ Dry eyes
➤ Jaw pain
➤ Headache
➤ Irritable bowel syndrome
➤ Bladder problems
➤ Poor concentration
➤ Depression or anxiety

Symptoms may be chronic, but they probably aren't constant: They may come and go, affected by weather changes, stress, physical activity—even the time of day. It's not unusual, for

INSTANT ACTION

■ Soothe aching muscles, tendons, and ligaments with a long, hot shower.

■ Apply a hot-water bottle or heating pad.

■ Take over-the-counter acetaminophen.

■ Get a massage for lingering relief of pain and better sleep.

■ Consider supplements of fish oil, or combinations of magnesium and malic acid.

example, to wake up achy and stiff, but feel more comfortable as the day wears on, only to start feeling worse again at night.

SELF-CARE STRATEGIES

Soothing warmth. To relieve the morning aches and stiffness that often accompany fibromyalgia, start your day with a hot shower. To use heat throughout the day, apply a hot-water bottle or heating pad to painful trigger points.

Better sleep habits. There's no magic solution to sleeping more soundly when you have fibromyalgia, but you should make sure you're not overlooking sleep robbers that are under your control. Go to bed and get up at the same times each day, lay off caffeine by midafternoon, wind down with some kind of bedtime ritual, and avoid alcohol at bedtime.

A vegetarian diet. Some studies suggest that going meatless relieves pain, eases stiffness, and improves sleep in people with fibromyalgia. Also consider eliminating food allergens such as corn, wheat, dairy, citrus, and sugar, which in some cases appear to make fibromyalgia symptoms worse. So-called elimination diets entail giving up potential offenders, then gradually reintroducing them one at a time to see if a particular food triggers more pain.

Exercise. Surprisingly, one of the best ways to relieve fibromyalgia's pain and fatigue is by exercising hard enough to get the heart pumping. Some experts go so far as suggesting deconditioned muscles may be a cause of fibromyalgia. Regular aerobic workouts reduce the number of tender points in fibromyalgia patients, according to a 2002 study published in the *British Medical Journal*. It found that fibromyalgia patients who took aerobics classes were far more likely to rate themselves much or very much better after three months than a similar group who took relaxation classes. Some exercisers improved so much, they no longer met the criteria for fibromyalgia. To ease into exercise:

➤ Choose a low-impact workout such as stationary cycling, walking, swimming, or water exercise.

➤ Start with just five minutes every other day if you're in a lot of pain or out of shape.

➤ Gradually work up to 30 to 60 minutes a day, four times a week.

CHECKLIST FOR RELIEF

✔ Self-Care Strategies

Heat	p. 89
Eye drops	
Vegetarian diet	
Eliminating food triggers	
Better sleep habits	p. 141
Aerobic exercise	p. 104
Spray and stretch	

✔ Medical Measures

Acetaminophen	p. 44
Antidepressants	p.136
Muscle relaxants	p.180
Anti-anxiety drugs	
Lidocaine injections	

✔ Complementary Options

Massage	p.100
Hypnosis	p. 80
Spinal manipulation	p.101
Acupuncture	p.113
SAMe	p.124
5-HTP	
Fish oil	
Magnesium and malic acid	

➤ Skip high-impact aerobic exercise and weightlifting for now—they may make discomfort from fibromyalgia worse.

Spray and stretch. Enlist a friend or family member to help you with "spray and stretch," a technique that can significantly ease pain from fibromyalgia. Your doctor or physical therapist can explain details of the method, which entails spraying a coolant such as ethyl chloride or Fluori-Methane over a painful area. Your partner then slowly stretches the targeted muscle, which—because it's been chilled—shouldn't hurt while it's being handled. Afterward your muscles feel more relaxed, have greater range of motion, and are less racked with pain—effects that last for days or even weeks.

Social support. Research suggests that support from family, friends, or even other patients can significantly ease symptoms of fibromyalgia. In one study, people with fibromyalgia reported improvement after participating in a group therapy program that invited significant others to participate, while also offering mind/body techniques and coping strategies to ease pain and handle the emotional burdens of having the condition.

MEDICAL MEASURES

OTC pain relievers. To relieve achiness from fibromyalgia, reach first for over-the-counter acetaminophen (Tylenol)—probably a better bet as a stand-alone drug than NSAIDs such as ibuprofen or naproxen. Reason: Fibromyalgia isn't caused by muscle or joint inflammation, which are the targets of NSAIDs—so there's no reason to risk NSAIDs' potential gastric side effects.

Antidepressants. Amitriptyline (Elavil or Endep), a tricyclic antidepressant, seems to reduce pain, relax muscles, and improve quality of sleep in people with fibromyalgia, though its effects may fade with continued use. Using an antidepressant, perhaps along with another medication, appears to reduce fibromyalgia in about 25 percent of patients.

Combination treatments. Doctors find that using the antidepressants amitriptyline and fluoxetine (Prozac) together seems more effective against fibromyalgia than either drug

---

FIGURING OUT FIBROMYALGIA

Fibromyalgia has only been defined since 1990, when the American College of Rheumatology laid down the criteria for a diagnosis. Before that, the syndrome went by a number of names: fibrositis, chronic muscle pain syndrome, psychogenic rheumatism, and tension myalgias. But arriving at what fibromyalgia is hasn't helped reveal its elusive cause. Among the proposed—but yet unproven—possibilities:

■ A genetic predisposition

■ Bacterial or viral infection

■ Spinal injury

■ Sleep deprivation

■ Emotional trauma

■ Psychological difficulties

■ Chemical changes in the brain

■ An abnormality in the sympathetic nervous system

alone. Other potentially effective combinations include fluoxetine and the muscle relaxant cyclobenzaprine (Flexeril), and the anti-anxiety drug alprazolam (Xanax) with ibuprofen.

Anesthetic injections. A more invasive (and thus controversial) approach is to inject lidocaine (Xylocaine) into tender points, which stops pain temporarily, but usually doesn't permanently end the cycle of pain and sleep loss.

COMPLEMENTARY OPTIONS

Mind/body techniques. Almost any stress-reduction technique can help you cope with the physical and mental frustrations of fibromyalgia, but some seem to be especially beneficial. Recent studies have found that:

➤ Regular massage treatments may offer longer-lasting relief than relaxation therapy. Patients getting either therapy felt less stressed and were in better moods immediately after their sessions in a 2002 study, but only the rubdown recipients had longer lasting effects—logging more hours of sleep, feeling less pain, and having fewer tender points.

➤ Hypnosis improved function and reduced fibromyalgia pain more effectively than physical therapy.

➤ Fibromyalgia patients treated with four weeks of spinal manipulation showed more improvement than those who took only medications. (Caution: Chiropractic techniques may not be safe for older people with severe symptoms.)

➤ People who got real acupuncture reported less pain and depression than those who received a sham treatment in which needles were placed randomly.

SAMe. S-adenosylmethionine, a substance produced from an amino acid and ATP, the body's main energy molecule, has been shown to reduce pain, fatigue, and depression from fibromyalgia. However, studies used injectable SAMe, which may have different effects than the oral supplement.

5-HTP. Early evidence suggests that 5-HTP (5-hydroxytryptophan, a form of another amino acid) may improve sleep and make tender points less sensitive.

Nutritional supplements. According to the National Institutes of Health, fish oil and combinations of magnesium and malic acid (a fruit extract) may also be effective.

READY RESOURCES

Fibromyalgia Network
P.O. Box 31750
Tucson, AZ 85751-1750
Phone: 800-853-2929
Website: www.fmnetnews.com

National Fibromyalgia Association
2238 N. Glassell St.
Suite D
Orange, CA 92865
Phone: 714-921-0150
Fax: 714-921-6920
Website: www.fmaware.org

National Fibromyalgia Partnership
140 Zinn Way
Linden, VA 22642-5609
Phone: 866-725-4404
Fax: 866-666-2727
Website:
www.fmpartnership.org

Everyone's intimately familiar with Mother Nature's call, but when you have interstitial cystitis, the urge to urinate becomes more of an unhappy holler as feelings of pressure and pain surround the bladder and pelvic area, compelling you to void up to 60 times a day. But while pain from interstitial cystitis can make it difficult to have sexual intercourse, ride in a car, or sit at a desk, symptoms usually don't get worse over time, and about half of patients go into remission, sometimes for years. During flare-ups, you can implement a number of strategies to control irritation and pain—and take back your life.

Understanding the Pain

To the 700,000 Americans who have interstitial cystitis (IC)—90 percent of whom are women—symptoms may seem like those of a urinary tract infection, or UTI. But while a UTI is a bacterial invasion that's easily treated with antibiotics, recurring IC is more mysterious.

With IC, the bladder wall becomes inflamed for unknown reasons. Usually, the inflammation takes the form of pinpoint-size hemorrhages called glomerulations, though about 5 to 10 percent of patients have cracks, scars, and star-shaped sores called Hunner's ulcers, an even more severe form of IC. The fuller the bladder, the greater the discomfort, so voiding provides a measure of relief—but the need to urinate seems almost constant, especially at night, when it's not unusual to get up 10 to 20 times. The tiresome nature of the condition can lead to exhaustion and depression, but some patients also report muscle and joint pain, migraines, allergic reactions, and gastrointestinal problems.

Researchers have several theories, none proven, regarding the underlying source of IC. These include:

➤ An as-yet undiscovered infectious agent
➤ An allergic reaction

INSTANT ACTION

■ Avoid caffeine, alcohol, carbonated drinks, and acidic juices.

■ Try not to eat spicy foods.

■ Don't smoke.

■ Start a diary of bathroom breaks, which you can use to build bladder control.

➤ A hormonal link

➤ An autoimmune disorder, in which the body's infection-fighting mechanisms turn against healthy tissue, perhaps following a bladder infection

➤ Leaks in the bladder's protective inner lining (the glycosaminoglycan, or GAG, layer) that allow toxins from urine to seep into the bladder wall

SELF-CARE STRATEGIES

The average age of IC diagnosis is about 40, but the on-again, off-again nature of the disease means you won't always be saddled with discomfort—especially if you take charge of your condition with steps ranging from changing your diet to taking drugs specially developed to fight this problem.

Bladder exercises. You can make IC more tolerable through a self-help technique known as bladder retraining, in which you schedule times for bathroom visits, gradually lengthening the time between voiding. This exercise in willpower strengthens the bladder muscle, which may weaken when frequent urination prevents it from fully distending. You might chart your daily plan and progress in a diary, and use relaxation or distraction when the urge to void comes before a scheduled bathroom break.

Modify your diet. Although the National Institute of Diabetes and Digestive and Kidney Diseases says there's no scientific evidence linking diet to interstitial cystitis, many doctors and patients believe the foods and beverages you ingest can affect the frequency and pain of urination. Steps that may help include avoiding substances known to stimulate the bladder, such as alcohol, caffeine, carbonated beverages, acidic juices, and spicy foods. Smoking and, of course, constantly sipping beverages also make you urinate more.

Practical help. If you seem to feel more miserable after you eat or drink a certain food or beverage, stop eating it for a while, then reintroduce it, to see if you feel better or worse. For example, some people believe artificial sweeteners make symptoms more intense; others blame rye or sourdough bread; still others point to dairy products, cured meats, nuts, or certain fruits or vegetables. If you suspect multiple foods to be a problem, elim-

CHECKLIST FOR RELIEF

✔ **Self-Care Strategies**
Bladder retraining
Eliminating bladder-stimulating foods
Controlling fluid intake
Identifying problem foods

✔ **Medical Measures**
Bladder distention
Bladder instillation
IC-specific drugs
NSAIDs   p. 41
Tricyclic antidepressants   p.136
Antihistamines
Removing ulcers
Enlarging bladder
Removing bladder
Sacral nerve root stimulation

✔ **Complementary Options**
TENS   p.102
Biofeedback   p. 78

inate only one type of food or beverage at a time to pinpoint those that seem to provoke the worst reactions. Just be sure to keep your overall diet varied and well-balanced to maintain general good health.

MEDICAL MEASURES

Expanding the bladder. Curiously, one of the techniques for finding interstitial cystitis—cytoscopy—actually makes some people feel better, at least temporarily. The reason: In order to see inside the bladder with a cytoscope (a tube about the size of a drinking straw), the doctor stretches the bladder with a liquid or gas, a process called distention. Experts speculate that pain relief comes from increasing the bladder's capacity, or that the procedure interferes with the bladder's transmission of pain signals. In fact, this diagnostic step is sometimes also considered a first step of medical treatment.

Bladder instillation. Also known as a bladder wash or bath, bladder instillation is a bit like distention: Using a narrow tube, or catheter, the bladder is filled with a solution such as dimethyl sulfoxide (DMSO, or Rimso-50), which is held for 10 to 15 minutes before being emptied. The drug penetrates the bladder wall to reduce inflammation and relax muscles, and it may prevent muscle contractions that lead to urinary pain, frequency, and urgency. You typically get treatments every week or two for six to eight weeks. Some patients learn to do the process themselves to save the time and cost of doctor's visits. In one study, more than 50 percent of patients experienced significant relief with DMSO. Treatment produces a strange but harmless side effect: a garlic-like taste and odor. Fortunately, breath and skin freshen after about three days. DMSO may also be used with heparin, another instilled drug, which may help repair problems in the bladder wall.

Oral medications. Pentosan polysulfate sodium (Elmiron), the first oral drug developed for IC, has been shown to improve symptoms in about one-third to one-half of patients. How it works isn't clear, but doctors believe it may fix defects in a leaky

GETTING TO THE BOTTOM OF IC

Before interstitial cystitis is finally diagnosed, most patients consult at least five physicians, including psychiatrists, over the course of four or more years. One reason: A number of other conditions must be ruled out, including uterine fibroids, endometriosis, ovarian cysts, pelvic inflammatory disease, vaginitis, bladder cancer, kidney stones, and sexually transmitted diseases, as well as prostate infections in men.

bladder lining, preventing the entrance of irritants in urine. Be patient for results, though: It can take up to six months to notice the drug's beneficial effects. Some IC experts believe the best pain relief is achieved by taking two oral medications. Small doses of tricyclic antidepressants (such as Elavil and Sinequan) help block pain, calm bladder spasms, and reduce inflammation, while antihistamines (such as Atarax) seem to help patients who also have allergies, migraines, or irritable bowel syndrome. Nonsteroidal anti-inflammatory drugs (NSAIDs) may ease pain that's either mild (over-the-counter types, such as Advil or Motrin) or more severe (prescription Celebrex or Vioxx).

Surgical solutions. Surgery for IC is considered a last resort, reserved for patients with disabling pain that's unrelieved by other treatments. Options include removing Hunner's ulcers by burning them with electricity or a laser (fulguration) or cutting them out (resection). The bladder may also be enlarged (augmentation) or, in cases where no other option seems to help, totally removed (cystectomy).

A surgical variation of transcutaneous electrical nerve stimulation (TENS), called sacral nerve root stimulation, shows promise as well. A device is implanted below the skin of the lower back, near the sacral nerve, and sends pulses to nerves involved in bladder function. It's usually used to treat bladder-control problems, and researchers who are now testing it as an IC treatment hope it may also help control the frequency and urgency of urination associated with this disease.

COMPLEMENTARY OPTIONS

Transcutaneous electrical nerve stimulation (TENS) appears to be particularly beneficial for IC discomfort, with symptoms improving or even disappearing (at least for a while) in more than half of patients who have Hunner's ulcers, and 26 percent who don't. Scientists aren't sure just how it works, but theorize that the mild electrical pulses increase blood flow to the bladder, strengthen pelvic muscles that help control the bladder, or trigger the release of pain-blocking substances.

Meanwhile, for some people with IC, using biofeedback to relax the pelvic floor muscles helps calm the spasms that lead to IC symptoms.

READY RESOURCES

Interstitial Cystitis Association
110 N. Washington St.
Suite 340
Rockville, MD 20850
Phone: 800-435-7422
Fax: 301-610-5308
Website: www.ichelp.org

National Institute of Diabetes and Digestive and Kidney Diseases
Office of Communications and Public Liaison, NIDDK
National Institutes of Health
Building 31, Room 9A04
31 Center Dr., MSC 2560
Bethesda, MD 20892-2560
Website: www.niddk.nih.gov

The name sounds emotional, as if your innards were capable of becoming annoyed and angry. Irritable bowel syndrome (IBS) was, in fact, once considered a psychological problem. Today, however, it's known to be a physical disorder that afflicts 10 to 20 percent of Americans. There's comfort in those numbers: Given the size of the problem, doctors have worked to find ways you can take charge of gastric pain and discomfort at home. Just as important, researchers have developed numerous drugs to take the edge off IBS—including a new generation of medications that, if used safely, offer even more hope for relief. And while emotions don't cause the disorder, you can put your mind to work to keep pain and discomfort from flaring.

Understanding the Pain

Once known as spastic colon or colitis, irritable bowel syndrome's unpleasant hallmarks are abdominal pain, diarrhea or constipation, bloating, and gas—the usual villains when food travels either too quickly or too slowly through your system. The underlying issue is the consistency of your stools. With IBS, they tend to be either too loose or too hard—often in alternating bouts of both.

IBS doesn't pose a serious health threat to your intestines or your body overall, but it can have a significant impact on daily life. "It's responsible for more absenteeism than any disorder other than the common cold," says Kevin Olden, M.D., associate professor of medicine at the Mayo Clinic in Scottsdale, Arizona. Symptoms often strike soon after eating, though sometimes you can't even finish a meal before cramping up or needing to make an urgent trip to the bathroom. For women, who are two to three times more likely to deal with IBS than men, symptoms often become worse around menstruation. But when-

INSTANT ACTION

■ Ease abdominal pain by relaxing in a warm bath or holding a hot-water bottle or heating pad on your stomach.

■ Put on loose-fitting clothes that don't press down on your gut.

■ Take an over-the-counter antidiarrheal to firm up loose stools.

■ Take a fiber supplement to help relieve constipation.

■ Chew an antacid to get rid of pain from gas and bloating.

ever you experience it, pain tends to settle in the lower abdomen, and can feel dull and aching or sharp and sudden. As with menstrual pain, some IBS sufferers find the discomfort to be mild and merely annoying, but for many others, the pain and bowel problems are severe and disruptive, making it difficult to attend social functions, carry on with regular work, or travel even short distances.

Though diet plays a role in triggering bouts, recent evidence suggests that IBS is caused by problems in the nerves that control contractions and sensations in the bowel. In a sense, multiple triggers are a blessing in disguise, giving you and your doctor a number of different approaches for easing pain and bringing discomforting bowel movements under control.

SELF-CARE STRATEGIES

Avoiding triggers. When you have IBS, it doesn't take much to send colon muscles into spasm, so substances that might not bother other people can easily irritate your gut. For preemptive pain control, it's best to avoid common culprits, such as chocolate, milk products, alcohol, caffeine, and high-fructose corn syrup. You should also steer clear of sugar-free desserts or candies made with sorbitol, a commonly used artificial sweetener, which is difficult to digest and has been known to trigger bouts of IBS.

Fiber. You don't need to swear off all sweet foods. Fruits such as figs, pears, and peaches all make good substitutes that provide an anti-IBS bonus: They're rich in fiber, which tends both to soften hard stools and firm up loose ones, easing the discomfort and pain that can come from on-again, off-again diarrhea and constipation. Just one caution: If your current diet is low in fiber, increase your intake of fresh produce, bran, or beans slowly. When the body's not used to it, fiber can make you gassy and may temporarily aggravate diarrhea. Introducing fiber over a period of weeks, however, allows your system to get used to it. A rule of thumb is to add 5 grams of fiber per day (about the amount in half a cup of kidney beans), but check with your doctor about what will work best for you.

Low-fat diet. Eating more fruits, vegetables, and beans has a third major benefit: All are low in fat, and eating them instead

CHECKLIST FOR RELIEF

✔ **Self-Care Strategies**

Low-fat diet
Fiber
Scheduled meals
Regular exercise   p. 71

✔ **Medical Measures**

Alosetron
Tegaserod maleate
Antispasmodics
Antidepressants   p.136
Antidiarrheals
Fiber supplements
Antacids

✔ **Complementary Options**

Biofeedback   p. 79
Meditation   p. 78
Deep breathing   p. 71
Hypnosis   p. 80
Progressive muscle
relaxation   p. 17
Cognitive behavioral therapy
Peppermint
Chinese herbs

IRRITABLE BOWEL SYNDROME
Ailments

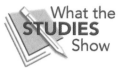
Doctors may be slow to diagnose irritable bowel syndrome, according to researchers at Vanderbilt University Medical Center in Nashville. They surveyed HMO participants about IBS symptoms and found that only 4 of 94 patients who met the criteria for the condition received a doctor's diagnosis during the previous year.

Patients share some of the blame for underdiagnosis of IBS: Epidemiological studies find that one-quarter to one-half of people with IBS symptoms don't seek healthcare.

of richer foods has immediate pain-protective effects. Fat in any form—meats, whole milk, butter, and even so-called heart-healthy oils such as olive oil—stimulates contractions in the colon. In fact, the speed and strength of cramping and other IBS symptoms after eating is directly related to how much fat is in your food, according to the National Institute of Diabetes and Digestive Disorders.

Meal management. Taking charge of your meal timing can help relieve pain and discomfort from both diarrhea and constipation, depending on which tends to bother you most. To avoid diarrhea, eating less at each meal—but eating more often—may ease cramping and bouts of loose stools. To sidestep constipation, eating three larger meals can help manage bowel movement by stimulating the muscle contractions that pass stools through your system.

Physical activity. Regular physical activity—about 30 minutes a day, almost every day—helps stimulate normal intestinal contractions, reducing constipation and diarrhea. A heart-pumping aerobic workout can also relieve stress that may help provoke symptoms.

MEDICAL MEASURES

New medications. In early 2000, the first of a new generation of drugs to treat IBS symptoms became available when the Food and Drug Administration approved alosetron (Lotronex), which works on the neurotransmitter serotonin to relax the colon, slow stool movement, and prevent diarrhea. It got off to a rocky start: In November 2000, the manufacturer voluntarily pulled the drug from the market after a few cases of serious side effects, such as ischemic colitis, an intestinal disorder, were reported. But in June 2002, the FDA allowed Lotronex to be sold again—with restrictions that minimize risks while taking best advantage of the drug's benefits. In 2002, the FDA also approved tegaserod maleate (Zelnorm), a drug that's ideal for short-term use in women with IBS-caused constipation.

Traditional treatments. If you don't fit gender and symptom requirements for new IBS drugs, your doctor can still draw from a wealth of time-tested treatments. These include antispasmodics such as dicyclomine and hyoscyamine (Levsin), which help relax intestinal muscles and relieve abdominal pain, and antidepressants such as tricyclic agents and selective serotonin reuptake inhibitors (SSRIs), which may be prescribed for severe cases of IBS pain.

OTC offerings. Several products on drugstore shelves may also help keep IBS symptoms in check, including antidiarrheals such as loperamide (Imodium and Kaopectate). Fiber supplements (Citrucel and Metamucil) may help reduce constipation, while antiflatulence medications such as simethicone (Gas-X and Mylicon) and antacids (Maalox, Mylanta, and Tums) help relieve gas and bloating.

COMPLEMENTARY OPTIONS

Relaxation techniques. Stress doesn't cause IBS symptoms, but it makes them worse, so relaxation techniques can help relieve your abdominal distress. Methods such as progressive muscle relaxation, meditation, deep breathing, and biofeedback may prove helpful. Studies suggest that hypnotherapy in which you imagine intestinal muscles becoming relaxed may be particularly beneficial for easing abdominal pain and bloating. Similarly, cognitive behavioral therapy can help you cope with the strain of chronic discomfort.

Peppermint. Research evidence suggests that peppermint, a natural antispasmodic, can help relax intestinal muscles. In one study, IBS sufferers who took an enteric-coated peppermint capsule before meals experienced less bloating, diarrhea, and abdominal pain. Not just any form of peppermint is beneficial: Uncoated capsules or peppermint tea may aggravate IBS, causing heartburn that makes symptoms worse.

Chinese herbs. The herbal formulas for coping with IBS that are found in health-food stores and on the Internet may be worth a try: A study published in *The Journal of the American Medical Association* found that people who took Chinese herbal blends for IBS fared better than those who took a placebo. However, don't use herbal preparations before first consulting your doctor and be sure to get your herbal formulas from reputable suppliers or stores.

READY RESOURCES

IBS Association
1440 Whalley Ave. #145
New Haven, CT 06515
Phone: 416-932-3311
Fax: 416-932-8909
Website:
www.ibsassociation.org

International Foundation for Functional Gastrointestinal Disorders
P.O. Box 170864
Milwaukee, WI 53217-8076
Phone: 414-964-1799
Fax: 414-964-7176
Website: www.iffgd.org

Ailments

Few people escape the pounding pain of an aching head: About 90 percent of us get headaches at one time or another, for various reasons—too much stress, too little sleep, a bout of feverish illness. For an estimated 45 million Americans, however, headaches hit with alarming frequency, causing ferocious pain that interferes with everyday life. But no matter what type of headache you're fighting, you can ease your agony with a combination of powerful medications that relieve the pain or counteract its cause. Beyond that, a wide range of nondrug treatments can soothe headache pain when it occurs or prevent it from flaring up.

Understanding the Pain

"Having a headache" isn't a single experience, but an array of different problems linked to the body's electrical network, muscles, and biochemistry. It's not always clear why headaches occur, but doctors divide them into a number of major categories:

Migraines. One of the most severe and debilitating forms of headache, migraines cause a relentless throbbing on one or both sides of the head that may continue for a few hours or as long as three days. Often accompanied by nausea, vomiting, and an oversensitivity to light, odors, and sound, migraines sometimes give sufferers a warning sign known as an aura, usually consisting of flickering or zigzagging lights or colors, a blind spot, a peculiar odor, or numbness. Close to 28 million Americans—about three-quarters of them women—suffer from migraines, sometimes as often as once or twice a week but usually less frequently. Many researchers believe migraines are caused by inherited cell abnormalities in the brainstem. A variety of triggers, including certain foods, stress, hunger, and sleeping too much or too little, may cause neurons to fire, awaken nerve pain, and inflame blood vessels.

INSTANT ACTION

- Gently press or massage your head to make flare-ups of pain more tolerable.

- Knead your neck, shoulders, and back to ease tension that can contribute to pain.

- Take a hot shower.

- Place a heating pad on your back to relieve pain-producing tightness.

- Apply an ice pack to your head to cool pain at the site.

- Take acetaminophen or aspirin products that are mixed with caffeine.

- Breathe deeply to ease tension and calm your nerves.

Cluster headaches. Most common in men, these headaches get their name from the fact that their intense, stabbing pain tends to flare up consistently over weeks or months at about the same time of the day or—most likely—night. A typical attack starts around one eye, which may become red and watery, then spreads to the side of the face. Pain usually ends after 30 to 45 minutes, only to repeat about 24 hours later. In some cases, more than one attack occurs in a day. After weeks or months of daily strikes, cluster headaches often mysteriously go into remission. No one yet knows what causes them, but research suggests that blood flow patterns or an abnormality in the brain's body clock may play a role.

Tension headaches. Two aspects of tension are at work in a typical episode of tension headache: Mental stress, which can trigger the pain, and a physical sensation like that of a belt tightening around the head. Most people have tension headaches every now and then, but for some people, they become chronic, occurring at least 15 times a month. Depression and anxiety can make pain more likely, but attacks can also be triggered by physical factors such as poor posture that strains head and neck muscles—for example, cradling a phone with your shoulder. Some tension headaches are brought on by other conditions, such as spinal arthritis or temporomandibular disorders.

SELF-CARE STRATEGIES

Self-massage. With any form of headache, using your hands to apply gentle, well-placed pressure may make the pain more bearable, at least temporarily. Don't stop with your throbbing temples, however: Knead your neck, shoulders, and back—areas where muscular tension can sometimes radiate upward, making headache pain worse.

Heat and cold. Taking a hot shower or applying moist heat to the back can help melt away a tension headache, while applying an ice pack to your head may help ease any type of ache. "It may be helpful to use both at the same time," suggests Christina Peterson, M.D., medical director of the Oregon Headache Clinic in Milwaukie. "Put heat on the neck to relax muscles, and ice on the head to relieve pain."

Diet dodges. At least a quarter of migraine sufferers find

CHECKLIST FOR RELIEF

✔ **Self-Care Strategies**
Self-massage
Heat and cold — p. 88
Avoid food triggers
Regular meals
Magnesium
Aerobic exercise — p.104

✔ **Medical Measures**
Aspirin
Acetaminophen — p. 44
Serotonin agonists
Ergotamine tartrate
Injected opioids — p. 54
Calcium channel blockers
Beta blockers
Antidepressants — p. 48
Anticonvulsants — p. 49
Pure oxygen
Corticosteroids — p. 44
Lithium

✔ **Complementary Options**
Biofeedback — p. 79
Meditation — p. 78
Deep breathing — p. 71
Imagery — p. 74
Behavioral therapy
Acupuncture — p.113
Feverfew

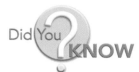

their headaches are triggered by certain foods and drinks, says Peterson. Common culprits to avoid include alcohol, cheese, cured meats, and pickles.

Regular meals. Eliminate the offenders, but don't skimp on eating other healthful foods—skipping meals may lead to low blood sugar, another possible headache trigger.

Magnesium. You may also want to supplement your diet with this mineral: Researchers believe that below-par levels of magnesium may contribute to migraine and cluster headaches.

Aerobic exercise. Regular aerobic exercise, which releases endorphins (natural painkillers), may also help keep headaches at bay. If you feel an impending headache, and you don't yet feel too ill, set out for an easy walk, ride a bike, or go for a swim—you may be able to contain the pain. Some sufferers of cluster headaches report that even more vigorous activity, such as jogging or running up and down stairs, can fend off an incoming attack.

MEDICAL MEASURES

OTC pain relievers. You can ease or end mild, occasional migraines or tension headaches with an early dose of aspirin or acetaminophen. For migraines, products that that also contain caffeine, such as Anacin or Excedrin, may be especially effective.

Triptans. Sumatriptan, zolmitriptan, almotriptan, and similar members of a recent class of drugs called serotonin agonists offer the most promise for relieving migraines. Triptans, which constrict dilated blood vessels and reduce inflammation, work best if taken at the start of an attack, but about a third of patients whose migraines are in full swing may also get relief. Sumatriptan (Imitrex) tablets seem to be especially helpful for women who suffer from menstrual migraines: In a 2002 study, almost 60 percent of women who took them for still-mild pain were headache-free two hours later. Because nausea can make it hard to keep pills down, some of these drugs come in alternative forms, such as a shot or nasal spray or a melt-under-the-tongue wafer. Another plus for triptans: They tend to produce fewer side effects such as nausea and high blood pressure than do traditional treatments for migraine.

Traditional treatments. Standard drug treatment for migraines has for 50 years centered on ergotamine tartrate

(Cafergot, Ergostat), the most common form of another class of drugs that constrict arteries and reduce inflammation. While their tendency to make nausea worse leads many doctors and patients to try triptans first, ergotamines are available in a variety of formulations and doses that can provide more options for patients who don't respond well to newer drugs.

Opioids. Narcotic medications are sometimes used in cases of severe headache pain that doesn't respond well to other treatments. Preferred formulations often mix opioids such as codeine with acetaminophen. Some doctors also recommend a nasal spray that works quickly and is less likely to cause or provoke nausea.

Preventives. If migraines strike at least three times a month, you may need a course of preventive medicine, ideally in small doses to avoid side effects from long-term use. Among the options are calcium channel blockers and beta blockers, drugs for high blood pressure that have a beneficial effect on blood vessels. Other preventive possibilities include antidepressants such as fluoxetine (Prozac) and MAO inhibitors, which may ease migraines by changing levels of the brain chemical serotonin, and anticonvulsants such as topiramate, which suppress abnormal firing of nerve cells.

Tension tamers. Chronic tension-type headaches may be treated—and prevented—with tricyclic antidepressants or MAO inhibitors. Muscle relaxants such as Flexeril and Soma, which actually work more on the brain to relieve pain than on the muscles of the body, may also help relieve tension headaches.

Cluster clearers. If you're blindsided by a cluster headache, take a deep breath—of pure oxygen. About 80 percent of patients find relief after inhaling pure oxygen for 10 to 15 minutes, which seems to help constrict blood vessels. But before you invest in an oxygen tank, reduction valve, and mask, try the technique in a doctor's office to make sure you're not among the few who don't respond to oxygen. Oral medications generally aren't helpful because cluster headaches usually subside naturally before the drugs can kick in. Shots or sprays of

ON THE REBOUND

If headache pain continues to grip you despite repeatedly popping over-the-counter analgesics, the problem may be your medication. Taking OTC painkillers 10 or more times a month can make nerve receptors crave the drug, leading to "rebound" headaches in which medication may cut pain briefly, but as soon as the drug wears off, you're hit with a new assault. At that point, taking more medication only makes things worse, says Christina Peterson, M.D., of the Oregon Headache Clinic in Milwaukie. Solution: Quit the drugs. Even if going cold turkey makes headaches seem worse at first, you'll likely feel better than ever after several weeks.

sumatriptan, however, may work quickly enough to hasten relief. Preventive drugs for cluster headaches include calcium channel blockers to keep blood vessels from constricting; corticosteroids (for short-term use) to reduce inflammation and swelling; divalproex sodium (Depakote), an anticonvulsant; and lithium. If you're in the middle of a batch of clusters, ergotamine may halt an imminent attack.

COMPLEMENTARY OPTIONS

Relaxation therapies. It may seem impossible to calm down when your head is pounding, but relaxation therapies such as meditation, deep breathing, imagery, and biofeedback can help diminish pain by controlling stress and muscle tension in the face, neck and shoulders. These methods seem most effective for tension headaches: According to research funded by the National Institute of Neurological Disorders and Stroke, people with tension headaches who combined stress relief with tricyclic antidepressants had fewer headaches than people who took medication alone.

Acupuncture. Both the National Institutes of Health and the World Health Organization affirm that acupuncture may reduce migraines and other headaches. Some patients find that incorporating acupuncture into their headache pain management plan allows them to reduce the amount of medication they need.

Feverfew. Though not well studied, some evidence suggests this time-honored herbal remedy helps prevent migraines in about half of patients—probably due to an active compound called parthenolide, which blocks inflammation.

BOTOX: A SHOT AT HEADACHE RELIEF

Botulinum toxin A—the nerve-deadening treatment best known as a wrinkle reducer—may also soothe headache pain, according to researchers in North Carolina. They recently injected Botox into the head or jaw muscles of 134 people who regularly suffer from a variety of headaches types, including migraines and tension headaches. Overall, 84 percent said each treatment led to substantial pain relief, on average rating the therapy 4.3 on a scale of 1 (no improvement) to 5 (excellent).

We tend to think of the neck as rising from the shoulders, but it's actually an extension of the spine—part of a single line that the shoulders cross like the bar of a T. Like the back, the neck is vulnerable to an array of torments, from acute muscle aches to chronic conditions that damage the above-the-shoulders structure doctors call the cervical spine. Almost everybody gets neck pain at some point—but almost nobody needs to endure it permanently. If you're like most people, your pain will eventually go away. If not, you can ease your discomfort significantly with any number of drugs, procedures, lifestyle changes, and physical therapies.

Understanding the Pain

Imagine a golf tee supporting a bowling ball, and you get an idea of what the cervical spine is up against: Its seven interlocking neck bones, or vertebrae, hold up the head, which weighs about 10 pounds. Unlike a static tee, however, the neck swivels and twists while supporting its heavy load. Given these mechanics, neck pain is almost inevitable from one cause or another, according to Richard A. Deyo, M.D., M.P.H., professor of medicine and health services at the University of Washington in Seattle. These pain initiators include:

Sprains and strains. These most common causes of neck pain often result from poor posture, such as hunching over a steering wheel or sleeping in an odd position. But more serious injuries occur with whiplash, a condition in which abrupt movement such as the impact of a car crash sends the head whipping in one direction while the body is thrown in another. The severe strain on muscles, tendons, or ligaments usually begins to hurt 12 to 24 hours after the injury, causing neck and shoulder pain, stiffness, and headache.

INSTANT ACTION

■ Put a butterfly pillow behind your head for side support of your neck while sitting in an easy chair.

■ When sleeping, use down-filled pillows instead of foam ones.

■ Apply cold or heat at the site of your pain.

■ Hold your neck in a neutral position to rest for short periods during stressful activities.

■ If necessary, wear a supportive neck collar for limited periods of time.

■ Do shoulder shrugs to ease tension and strengthen neck muscles.

Disk disorders. After about four decades of wear and tear, the jellylike disks that provide cushioning between the vertebrae start to dry out. Disks that herniate—that is, allow the inner core to protrude through the disk's tough outer covering—can irritate neighboring nerves, causing pain that can reach across the shoulder and down the arm. (Cervical disk problems can also result from sudden injuries.) Bony growths called spurs may aggravate the condition by pressing painfully on nerves or causing a narrowing of the cervical canal that holds the spinal cord.

Arthritis. The most common form of arthritis, osteoarthritis, is a degenerative joint disease that causes the spine to grow more rigid and makes the neck feel stiff and sore, a condition known as cervical spondylosis.

Other conditions. Neck pain can occur with a wide variety of diseases and conditions ranging from acute illnesses such as the flu to chronic problems including a neuromuscular disorder called wryneck, or torticollis, a condition that causes painful spasms on one side of the neck.

SELF-CARE STRATEGIES

Cold and heat. Both ice packs and heating pads can relieve neck pain, though which works best differs from one person to the next. As a rule, ice is most effective for acute injuries because the cold both dulls pain and reduces swelling or inflammation. Apply a bag of ice wrapped in a cloth or a cold gel pack (available in pharmacies) for no more than 15 or 20 minutes at a time. Longer-term pain may respond best to the relaxing effects of heat treatment, which, in addition to pads or hot-water bottles, can include hot baths or showers.

Pillows. To provide the cervical spine with comfortable support, especially in the evening, when some people find neck pain to be worse, try using a butterfly pillow when sitting on a sofa or easy chair. These pillows have cushy "wings" that gently support the neck at each side while the back of the neck rests against a pad. In bed, replace foam rubber pillows with pillows filled with down, which molds better to the shape of your head and neck, providing more consistent and comfortable support.

Posture control. You'll experience less pain if you keep the cervical spine properly aligned. Try to keep your ear, shoulder, and hip in a straight line on each side whether you're standing, sitting, or lying down. Nurture your neck when you're on the go or at work by not overloading shoulder bags, hunching forward in the driver's seat when visibility is poor, or cradling the phone between your neck and shoulder.

Back sleeping. Avoid sleeping on your side or stomach, which twists the neck out of alignment and can aggravate pain. Instead, sleep on your back with your head facing the ceiling, which keeps the entire spine straight and puts less pressure on the neck.

A stabilizing collar. Wearing a support collar (available from medical supply stores) around your neck can help ease pain by keeping the cervical spine stable and properly aligned while allowing muscles to be relatively relaxed. Consider it a temporary fix, however: Using a collar for more than about 10 days can cause neck muscles to become weaker and lose mobility, which ultimately makes pain worse.

Neck moves. Simple exercises that work the neck and shoulders may both help relieve neck pain you have right now and prevent future discomfort. An orthopedist or physical therapist can recommend stretching and strengthening exercises that are best for you. One possible example: From an upright position, shrug your shoulders up toward your neck as far as you can, hold for several seconds, then slowly relax.

MEDICAL MEASURES

Analgesics. Nagging neck pain can usually be appeased, at least for a while, with nonsteroidal anti-inflammatories (NSAIDs), available either over the counter (aspirin, Motrin, Aleve) or by prescription. If the drugs cause gastrointestinal distress, ask your doctor to prescribe COX-2 inhibitors, (Celebrex, Vioxx, Bextra), NSAIDs that are gentler on the stomach. Pain due to overly tense muscles can be eased with muscle relaxants that spur the nervous system to make muscles loosen up. Antidepressants and anti-anxiety drugs can help limit the transmission of neck pain through the nervous system. Corticosteroids may sometimes be prescribed for severe pain, though concerns about side effects limit how long they're used,

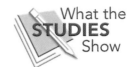
What the **STUDIES** Show

Surgery appears to offer no special benefit for people with cervical spondylosis (degeneration of the vertebrae in the neck), according to a report in the journal *Spine*. A review of studies found that while surgery might initially be more effective than physical therapy or cervical collars for reducing pain, after a year, patients fared equally well whether or not they'd been operated on.

READY RESOURCES

American Academy of Orthopaedic Surgeons
6300 N. River Rd.
Rosemont, IL 60018-4262
Phone: 800-346-2267; 847-823-7186
Fax: 847-823-8125
Website: www.aaos.org

Spine-health.com
1840 Oak Ave.
Suite 112
Evanston, IL 60201
Website:
www.spine-health.com

SpineUniverse.com
621 N.W. 53rd St.
Suite 240
Boca Raton, FL 33487
Website:
www.spineuniverse.com

with a typical course of oral medication running a week to 10 days, and injection therapies separated by a week.

Traction. This non-invasive mechanical treatment, in which you wear a device that uses a pulley system to raise the head and ease strain on the cervical spine, can bring speedy relief lasting hours or even days for some forms of neck pain.

Surgery is usually a last resort for neck pain, but may be necessary to relieve the pain, numbness, and weakness from nerve or spinal cord compression caused by a herniated disk or bony spur. Options include:

➤ Anterior or posterior cervical diskectomy, in which doctors make an incision in the front or back of the neck, enlarge the nerve opening, and remove the disk and any spurs.

➤ Posterior hemilaminectomy, in which surgeons enter the back of the neck to remove bone and ligaments as well as disk material.

COMPLEMENTARY OPTIONS

TENS. Some patients may find relief using transcutaneous electrical nerve stimulation (TENS), which sends tiny, pain-relieving electrical impulses through electrodes placed on the aching area.

Relaxing regimens. To relieve stress-related pain from tensed neck and shoulder muscles, try relaxation exercises such as progressive muscle relaxation, deep breathing, and meditation.

Manipulation. Pain in the spine is one of the conditions for which chiropractic is best supported by research. If you seek hands-on help through spinal manipulation, however, be sure to seek out a properly trained and licensed practitioner. "Manipulation of the neck poses greater risk of injury than manipulation of the low back," notes Deyo.

Acupuncture. You won't aggravate neck pain with needle therapy: The neck may be treated by stimulating points in the feet. The effectiveness of acupuncture for neck pain is not well established, but some patients find it provides relief. If you don't get results after six treatments, assume it's not working for you.

An old saw has it that "ulcers aren't caused by what you eat, but by what's eating you." It turns out that the original message of this saying—stress causes ulcers—is untrue. Now we know that bacteria are behind most peptic ulcers. Yet something is indeed eating you: stomach acid, which washes over sensitive sores created by germs boring into your gut. In one sense, this is good news: Today's ulcer treatments not only contain the pain, they can actually cure the problem. With the right therapy, complemented by lifestyle measures, you can be free of ulcer unpleasantness in relatively short order.

Understanding the Pain

At one time, peptic ulcers were blamed on spicy foods and stressful lives. Then about 20 years ago two Australian doctors revolutionized this view by discovering that people with ulcers tend to be infected by *Helicobacter pylori,* a spiral-shaped bacterium. Normally, *H. pylori* loiters peacefully in the stomach's protective mucous layer. But in about one out of six infected people, the bacterium for unknown reasons begins to damage this natural shield, leaving the stomach or intestinal lining vulnerable to caustic digestive acids and further bacterial damage. A peptic ulcer is the painful result.

"Peptic" means "pertaining to digestion," and peptic ulcers can appear throughout the digestive tract—for example, gastric ulcers occur in the stomach, and duodenal ulcers are found in the small intestine. All usually produce a dull, gnawing pain, often when the stomach is empty. This pain is sometimes accompanied by symptoms such as heartburn, nausea, and bloating. Less commonly, ulcer sufferers may develop sharp, constant pain and bloody or black stools or vomit. These are signs that the ulcer may have perforated the stomach or duodenal wall, broken a blood vessel, or obstructed the path of food—all of which demand immediate medical attention.

INSTANT ACTION

■ Take an antacid to relieve gastrointestinal pain.

■ Munch on fiber-rich fruits and vegetables to possibly speed healing.

■ Eat a few times a day to limit the flow of pain-producing acid.

■ Trust your gut. If a particular food makes you feel ill, avoid it.

PEPTIC ULCER

While the incidence of peptic ulcers appears to be decreasing, they're still common, affecting up to 10 percent of Americans at some point in their life. But thanks to a greater understanding of the condition, most ulcers can be readily cured with a two-pronged approach that kills bacteria and reduces acid.

SELF-CARE STRATEGIES

Protective nutrients. Even if foods are no longer thought to cause ulcers, some researchers say eating a diet rich in fiber may keep new ulcers from forming and reduce pain by helping existing ones heal. Fiber is thought to enhance the secretion of mucin, a component of protective mucus in the gut. Fiber-rich fruits and vegetables seem to be particularly helpful, possibly because the vitamin A found in produce such as yams also enhances mucin production. Other nutrients thought to have similar effects include vitamin E and zinc.

Flavonoids. Apples, cranberries, celery, onions, red wine, and tea may also be valuable for successfully fighting ulcers. All are rich in flavonoids, natural chemicals that appear to inhibit the growth of *H. pylori*.

Three square meals. A few medium-size meals seem to provoke fewer symptoms than frequent small meals. Try to avoid having a bedtime snack, which may boost acid flow and cause pain to flare during the night.

Judicious drinks. Coffee—regular or decaf—spurs the production of stomach acid, as do soft drinks and citrus juices. While no research proves a link between these beverages and ulcers, some researchers do say that drinking more than three cups of coffee a day may leave you more vulnerable to damage by *H. pylori*.

Potential pain aggravators. Although studies exonerate spicy foods from playing a role in ulcers, it still makes sense to avoid dietary items if they seem to irritate the stomach. Triggers for pain can vary from one person to the next, but potential offenders may include black pepper, chili powder, chocolate, peppermint, tomatoes, fatty foods, and dairy products. And while smoking and excessive drinking also have no clear connection with ulcers, they certainly don't help. For example, nicotine both increases stomach acid output and boosts the acid's strength.

MEDICAL MEASURES

The triple threat. The best treatment consists of what's called triple therapy: two drugs to attack the bugs plus another one to reduce acid. It's a demanding regimen, requiring up to 20 pills a day, but the course of treatment is usually short (two weeks) and effective a remarkable 90 percent of the time. (A less intensive, but less effective alternative plan called dual therapy consists of only one antibiotic and an acid suppressor.) The three prongs may include:

➤ **Antibiotics** to kill *H. pylori*. These include amoxicillin (Amoxil), clarithromycin (Biaxin), metronidazole (Flagyl), and tetracycline (Achromycin).

➤ **Acid blockers.** "These help relieve pain and also enhance the action of the antibiotic," says James Scheiman, M.D., associate professor of gastroenterology at the University of Michigan in Ann Arbor. Doctors often prescribe H2 blockers, which suppress the production of histamine, a substance that stimulates acid secretion. Available both over the counter and by prescription, H2 blockers include cimetidine (Tagamet), famotidine (Pepcid), nizatidine (Axid), and ranitidine (Zantac).

➤ **Proton pump inhibitors.** These alternatives to acid blockers shut down the mechanism that pumps acid into the

Ailments

stomach. Prescription-only proton pump inhibitors include lansoprazole (Prevacid), omeprazole (Prilosec), and rabeprazole (Aciphex).

OTC additions. Some regimens also include preparations that may be as close as your own medicine cabinet, such as bismuth subsalicylate (Pepto-Bismol). This time-honored treatment for stomach upset both coats the stomach lining and kills *H. pylori*. Antacids (Maalox, Mylanta, Tums), which neutralize stomach acid (but don't block its secretion), may also be used for fast pain relief.

COMPLEMENTARY OPTIONS

Licorice. In the form of deglycyrrhizinated licorice (DGL), this best-known (and probably most effective) complementary treatment for ulcers is thought to promote production of substances that protect the gut. Several studies have suggested that DGL may be even more effective than antacids for relieving ulcer pain. It has not, however, been shown to kill *H. pylori*, so it's not a real cure.

Relaxation methods. Some experts believe that anecdotal evidence is strong enough to support a link between stress and ulcers: Lab animals subjected to physical exhaustion or loud noises get ulcers. Even if stress doesn't cause ulcers, it can probably aggravate pain from an existing case. Stress-relieving methods such as deep breathing and progressive muscle relaxation can help temper tension.

ROMANCE AND RE-INFECTION

If you've successfully completed an ulcer-killing course of antibiotics, go ahead and give your significant other a kiss on the lips to celebrate. Even if he or she carries the bacterium (but, unlike you, never developed an ulcer), your partner's germs aren't likely to infect you again, according to a 2002 study. Researchers in Spain examined ulcer patients who'd been cured, then re-infected later, and looked at their partners as well. DNA tests revealed that even if the healthy spouses also tested positive for *H. pylori*, they carried different strains than their partners did—suggesting they didn't pass on ulcer-causing bugs by exchanging kisses.

Peripheral neuropathy—the broad term for a group of painful disorders involving the peripheral nervous system—was once considered an inevitable consequence of having diabetes. Groundbreaking research in recent years, however, has shown that damage from this top cause of peripheral neuropathy can be dramatically offset with lifestyle changes. And pain from nerve damage that's already occurred—no matter what the cause—can be addressed with treatments that attack the problem on multiple fronts.

Understanding the Pain

More than 2 million Americans have some form of neuropathy, though the exact nature of what they experience varies according to what type of nerves are affected and what caused them to be damaged:

Sensory nerves. When sensory nerves have been harmed, common symptoms include tingling and numbness—along with sharp, burning, or freezing pain, especially in extremities such as the hands and feet. Sometimes, nerves become ultra sensitive so that even a slight touch (such as the brush of a bed sheet—symptoms often get worse at night) can cause excruciating agony.

Motor nerves. When motor nerves suffer damage, muscles may get weaker.

Autonomic nervous system (ANS). The ANS, which controls the body's involuntary responses, may become impaired, resulting in symptoms such as sluggish digestion, sexual dysfunction, and difficulty controlling bladder function.

Sometimes neuropathy results from an injury or repetitive action that puts pressure on a single nerve—for example, typing for long periods on a computer or using crutches. In such cases, however, nerves are usually more vulnerable to damage in the first place due to an underlying disease. The most common of these is diabetes, which causes nerve damage in about 60 per-

INSTANT ACTION

■ Distract pain signals by applying a heat cream containing capsaicin, giving yourself a vibrating massage, or soaking your feet.

■ Consider taking a supplement of possibly nerve-saving alpha-lipoic acid or gamma-linolenic acid.

■ Eat smaller meals to ease digestive discomfort and control blood sugar if you have diabetes.

■ Appropriate exercise will provide better blood flow and muscle strength.

cent of cases. It's not entirely clear how diabetes harms nerves, but high blood sugar appears to hinder transmission of electrical impulses, rob nerves of oxygen by blocking circulation, and damage nerves' protective sheathing. But neuropathy can also have a range of other causes, such as autoimmune diseases (including rheumatoid arthritis), thyroid problems, exposure to toxins, and bacterial or viral infections.

Nixing Neuropathy

If you have a disease like diabetes that makes you vulnerable to peripheral neuropathy, it's important to be alert to symptoms, which are often subtle. Flare-ups of neuropathy can be tough to detect, but catching them early improves your chances of staving off or slowing further damage and pain. Don't be faked out if tingling, numbness, or burning seem to get better on their own: Such sensations often come and go, or swing from mild to more severe. Be especially on guard for symptoms that occur at night or in the feet, which are often affected first.

SELF-CARE STRATEGIES

Control blood sugar. If you have diabetes, studies have shown that keeping blood sugar low—often solely through lifestyle measures such as controlling calorie intake and getting the right amount of exercise—can reduce risks of developing further nerve damage by a whopping 60 percent.

Mind your B's. In some cases, neuropathy and the pain it causes are fostered by nutritional deficiencies, particularly of B vitamins such as B_6 and B_{12}, both of which are involved with nerve function. You can get vitamin B_6 from foods such as avocados, bananas, pork, potatoes, and fish such as tuna, while B_{12} is available from foods such as chicken, beef, and a variety of seafood. If you suffer from a B deficiency, talk to your doctor about taking a supplement.

Manage meal sizes. If you suffer from gastroparesis—a common, uncomfortable gastrointestinal condition caused when damaged nerves make digestion slow down—try eating smaller, more frequent meals or softer foods to ease the load on your gut.

Practical help. One of the greatest dangers with peripheral neuropathy is damage to the feet, which are especially vulnerable because deadened nerves can make you oblivious to injuries. Left unguarded or untreated, damaged feet are susceptible to further pain, infections, festering sores, and even amputation. To minimize damage:

➤ **Go over feet** with your eyes and hands at least once a day for blisters, cuts, bruises, cracking, peeling, areas that are unusually red or pale, or any other evidence of damage.

➤ **Keep shoes on.** Footwear protects against seemingly innocuous (but potentially devastating) injuries from blows, abrasion, or sharp objects. When outdoors, avoid going barefoot—even at the beach, where it's better to at least wear flip-flops, sandals, or clogs.

➤ **Clean carefully.** To keep feet free of fungal or bacterial infections, wash them every day using lukewarm water. Blot feet dry rather than rubbing, and be sure to dry thoroughly between toes to discourage fungal growth. Follow up by applying a moisturizing cream to prevent cracking.

➤ **Change footwear.** Put on clean socks at least once a day (more often if your feet sweat a lot), making sure they don't abrade by bunching up or rubbing skin with seams. Try to have at least two pairs of shoes that you can don on alternate days to give each pair a day to air out between wearings.

MEDICAL MEASURES

NSAIDs. Aspirin, ibuprofen, and other nonsteroidal anti-inflammatories—along with acetaminophen—can help relieve mild pain associated with peripheral neuropathy. As symptoms become more severe, however, you may require stronger medication, beginning with prescription NSAIDs.

Psychotropic drugs. For mild to moderately severe pain, doctors may prescribe antidepressants such as amitriptyline (Elavil), nortriptyline (Pamelor), desipramine (Norpramin), and imipramine (Tofranil), which have been shown to have analgesic effects, particularly with neuropathic pain. The same is true for anticonvulsant drugs such as carbamazepine (Tegretol), gabapentin (Neurontin), and phenytoin (Dilantin).

Drugs for secondary problems. Other medications may be used to combat specific conditions that can arise from neuropathy, including sildenafil (Viagra) for sexual dysfunction and

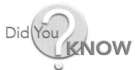
Did You KNOW

There's more than one type of neuropathy. The most common type, polyneuropathy ("poly" referring to "many"), affects multiple nerves throughout the body, but is often concentrated in the long peripheral nerves of the arms and legs, primarily causing sensation-disrupting symptoms such as pain or tingling. Another type, mononeuropathy ("mono" meaning "one"), affects a single nerve or set of nerves, so symptoms tend to concentrate in one area, typically within the muscles.

PERIPHERAL NEUROPATHY

Ailments

PERIPHERAL PRIMER

Consider all that healthy nerves do for you, and you get a sense of what can go wrong when you have peripheral neuropathy. Normally, the peripheral nerves—that is, nerves not part of the brain and spinal cord (which comprise the central nervous system)—serve a variety of functions by conducting electrical impulses through areas outside the central core of the body. These functions include providing sensation, moving your muscles, and controlling certain automatic functions such as digestion, blood pressure, and sweating. When peripheral nerves become damaged, a range of problems can develop—and pain is one of the most common.

various medications that fight high blood pressure and gastric problems. One drug used to treat irregular heart rhythms, mexiletine (Mexitil), can also help relieve certain types of pain.

Topical treatments. Topical ointments containing capsaicin (Capzasin, Zostrix), a compound found in hot peppers, relieve pain by interfering with signals that nerve cells send to the brain. Lidocaine patches release a local anesthetic onto the painful area.

COMPLEMENTARY OPTIONS

Neuropathic pain can be difficult to treat, and alternative treatments should never be used in place of a doctor's care. Still, when other treatments haven't worked, some complementary therapies may be worth trying.

Acupuncture appears to help in some cases of neuropathic pain, presumably by eliciting a response from the nerve pathways involved with pain.

Magnet therapy has had mixed results for treating pain, but some of the most promising results have been seen in research of neuropathic pain in people with diabetes.

Alpha-lipoic acid (ALA) and gamma-linolenic acid (GLA). Research on the role of these two supplements, produced naturally in the body, is limited and far from conclusive, but some studies suggest ALA reduces neuropathic pain, while GLA may help nourish nerves.

POSTHERPETIC NEURALGIA

Most adults can recall having chicken pox—once viewed as a childhood rite of passage before a vaccine arrived on the scene in the 1990s. But each year, up to one million adults are painfully reminded that the herpes zoster (or varicella zoster) virus that causes chicken pox can return with a vengeance as shingles. About a fifth of these patients develop a lingering nerve pain known as postherpetic neuralgia. Though neuropathic pain can be difficult to treat, don't ever feel you're stuck with it: A growing number of pain-relief options can tame the torment—until PHN naturally clears up on its own.

Understanding the Pain

The cause of PHN pain is clear: While dormant, the herpes zoster virus travels along nerves to an area near the spinal cord known as the dorsal root ganglia. Once reactivated (usually when immunity is lowered due to illness or stress), it spreads to nerve endings and travels up to the skin, causing shingles—a condition that creates painful blisters, usually on one side of the torso. The rash generally heals after several weeks, but with PHN, aching, throbbing, itching, burning, stabbing, or shooting pain persists for months—or even years. The affected area can become so sensitive that even the slight pressure of clothing, bed linens, or a gentle breeze can cause excruciating pain.

The risk of PHN increases with advancing age, especially among people whose nerves already work poorly due to diabetes or old age. The worse the kickoff case of shingles is, the more likely it will turn into PHN. While not all cases of PHN can be prevented, early evidence suggests that the varicella vaccine, available since 1995 and recommended for children, may also help reduce the severity of shingles and the risk of PHN in adults.

INSTANT ACTION

■ Put on comfortable clothes made of natural fibers such as cotton.

■ Take an over-the-counter analgesic such as acetaminophen or an NSAID as a first step to quelling pain.

■ For open herpes zoster sores, apply soothing calamine lotion.

■ For sores that have crusted over, redirect pain by rubbing on cream containing capsaicin.

■ Apply ice to the affected area.

■ Take deep breaths and use imagery to relax and try moving pain to the back of your mind.

POSTHERPETIC NEURALGIA
Ailments

Postherpetic neuralgia doesn't usually go on indefinitely: Less than a quarter of patients still have pain six months after the herpes zoster shingles eruption, and less than one in 20 has pain after a year. But don't just wait it out: Studies find that PHN responds far better to treatment that starts early, preferably within 30 days of when a shingles rash clears. Better yet, treating the virus during the shingles phase lowers the risk of PHN developing at all. Once you have PHN, however, there are a number of ways to minimize the pain.

SELF-CARE STRATEGIES

Natural fibers. To minimize pain from hypersensitivity of the skin, try dressing in clothing made from natural fibers such as cotton or linen, which may be less irritating than artificial fibers such as polyester or acrylics.

Ice. Applying ice to the affected area may relieve pain, at least temporarily. To ease initial contact with the skin, wrap ice bags, gel packs, or packs of frozen vegetables in a soft, clean cloth of natural fibers.

Topical ointments. Smoothing on topical creams can help ease pain at the surface of the skin. What you use depends on the condition of your varicella eruption. Start with soothing calamine lotion if you still have open lesions. After sores have crusted over, however, you can turn to ointments containing capsaicin (Zostrix), the oily chemical that gives hot peppers their bite. Though it can initially produce more irritation, capsaicin is the only FDA-approved treatment specifically for PHN because it's been shown to reduce pain by depleting nerve fibers of substance P, a pain-related peptide. Applied three to five times a day, capsaicin cream dulls pain after a few days to a week.

MEDICAL MEASURES

Skin patch. In 1999 the U.S. Food and Drug Administration approved a new treatment for PHN: the lidocaine patch (Lidoderm). It contains a pain-numbing solution (the type used by dentists) that penetrates the skin and reaches affected nerves, but doesn't enter the bloodstream, which keeps side effects to a minimum. Each patch is about the size of an adult's hand, and up to three at a time may be applied to the painful area. The patches stay in place for up to 12 hours, then are removed for 12 hours. Most patients get relief within a week or two.

Psychotropic drugs. Oral medication for PHN may start with gabapentin (Neurontin), an anticonvulsant that recently proved safe and effective in a large study of PHN patients, who reported less pain, improved sleep, and better moods when using the drug. Previously, tricyclic antidepressants such as nortriptyline topped the list of PHN drugs, and they continue to hold a high place on the roster of PHN pain-alleviating medications. Studies confirm their benefits for PHN, but relief usually comes slowly, as typical treatment begins with very low doses that are slowly increased to more effective levels.

Opioids. Though opioids are generally considered a last-resort option for PHN due to fears of side effects, mental impairment, and potential addiction, research published in late 2002 suggests the role of narcotics should be reconsidered. In a study of 76 patients with postherpetic neuralgia, researchers at Johns Hopkins University found that opioids relieved pain even better after eight weeks than gold-standard antidepressants, while causing no problems with cognitive function or dependence. And while opioids cause side effects such as nausea and constipation, patients in the study preferred them for pain over other treatments.

OTC painkillers. Analgesics such as acetaminophen (Tylenol) and nonsteroidal anti-inflammatories such as ibuprofen (Advil, Motrin, Nuprin) may have some effect on pain from PHN, but their benefits are far from dramatic. More often, these agents are used with stronger opioid painkillers to make the opioids more effective.

Invasive actions. Sympathetic nerve blocks, which involve injecting a local anesthetic into damaged nerves, may be tried if

PREEMPTIVE PAIN RELIEF

The quicker you are on the draw, the better you can quell PHN pain. That's the idea behind antiviral drugs that fight the herpes zoster virus directly. Taken early (ideally within 72 hours of a shingles outbreak), drugs such as acyclovir (Zovirax), valacyclovir (Valtrex), and famciclovir (Famvir) have been shown to shorten the duration of a herpes zoster eruption. Valacyclovir appears to be especially effective at cutting time spent suffering later from postherpetic neuralgia. Depending on which medication you use, antiviral drugs may be given orally or intravenously (sometimes along with a corticosteroid such as prednisone) and are generally well tolerated, though side effects can include gastrointestinal problems and headache. Unfortunately, once PHN has set in, these drugs provide no added benefit and aren't used for treatment.

POSTHERPETIC NEURALGIA
Ailments

READY RESOURCES

VZV Research Foundation
40 E. 72nd St.
New York, NY 10021
Phone: 800-472-8478
Fax: 212-861-7033
Website:
www.vzvfoundation.org

other less invasive measures are unsuccessful. However, they offer no guarantee of success, and when relief is attained, it seldom lasts long. Surgical procedures such as nerve ablation and spinal cord stimulation may provide great relief for a few patients, but are relatively risky and seldom recommended.

COMPLEMENTARY OPTIONS

TENS. Some researchers report that transcutaneous electrical nerve stimulation helps at least some PHN patients, and TENS is also sometimes used to treat shingles. But others find that the tingling sensations from this electrode treatment provide little comfort. Consider TENS one of many steps you can try to minimize your pain, but continue looking for other options if it doesn't work.

Mental control. Like other people with chronic pain, PHN patients may benefit from techniques that use the mind to cope with the body's pain. Among the most promising are:

➤ Biofeedback, which can help you recognize and soothe stress that can make PHN pain more difficult to bear

➤ Cognitive behavioral therapy, which helps some patients tame PHN pain through encouraging self-made statements such as "I've coped so far, and I'll continue to do so in the future"

➤ Hypnosis, which, if you're susceptible to hypnotic suggestion, can take your mind away from pain

Acupuncture. Spurred by its long traditional use for chronic pain, some postherpetic neuralgia patients say this ancient Chinese therapy helps relieve the pain of PHN, though what limited research has been done on PHN suggests it may be of limited use.

Vitamins. High doses of vitamin E—1000 to 1800 IU a day—may reduce the risk of PHN pain in shingles sufferers. Vitamin C, in doses of 1000 mg a day, may promote healing.

People often make light of PMS, joking about cravings—and ravings—that strike monthly like clockwork. But if you're among the 80 percent of menstruating women who suffer from premenstrual syndrome, you know it's about more than chocolate and churlishness: PMS can cause serious pain and discomfort ranging from bloating and breast tenderness to sore muscles and joints, headache, or nausea. But even if PMS is no laughing matter, there's reason to smile: You needn't accept monthly pain as an unfortunate fact of life—a common response, as indicated by a recent survey that found women with the most severe PMS were the least likely to seek help. Believe it: You can find relief from PMS. With the right treatment, you could be virtually PMS-free within three months.

Understanding the Pain

Researchers attribute some 150 different symptoms to PMS, many of which cause or exacerbate pain—including diarrhea, constipation, and gas, along with "softer" symptoms such as mood swings, appetite changes, clumsiness, and fatigue. So, while many women share the monthly misery of PMS, your symptoms—and how long you suffer from them—are likely to be different from the next woman's.

Whatever the nature of your experience, about 40 percent of PMS sufferers find pain and other monthly physical or emotional upsets unpleasant enough to make daily routines and relationships more difficult. Yet, as a rule, women soldier on, with several studies showing that (contrary to popular belief) premenstrual troubles don't hinder a woman's ability to actually carry out tasks. The exception is an estimated 3 to 8 percent of women who have a severe form of

INSTANT ACTION

■ Start taking pain relievers a week before your period starts, to fight headaches, backaches, and sore muscles.

■ Soothe cramps with a heating pad or warm bath.

■ Eat food with fiber to fend off constipation.

■ Put on a bigger bra to ease breast tenderness.

■ Take a diuretic to relieve discomfort from bloating.

■ Take a nonsteroidal anti-inflammatory drug such as naproxen for cramping and headache.

■ Challenge negative thinking to make pain more bearable.

PREMENSTRUAL SYNDROME
Ailments

PMS that warrants its own category: premenstrual dysphoric disorder, or PMDD. These women suffer from at least five largely emotional symptoms (including depression) that can make pain more difficult and are severe enough to be disabling.

With PMS, there's always light at the end of the tunnel: Symptoms naturally subside after about age 35 and end completely at menopause. But there's no need to wait. Even women with severe PMS can find a measure of relief through lifestyle changes, medication, or an unusually wide variety of herbal remedies.

SELF-CARE STRATEGIES

Recordkeeping. You'll be better able to relieve pain and other symptoms if you have a sure-handed understanding of how your monthly period progresses. Note symptoms and when they occur in a journal for at least three cycles, which can help you and a doctor determine the best course of action for your particular case.

Heat. To help relieve abdominal cramps, sit in a tub of warm water two or three times a day, when possible, or apply heat with a hot-water bottle, heating pad, or thick towel dampened with hot water.

Complex carbohydrates. Eating foods rich in complex carbohydrates (as opposed to simple sugars) helps relieve discomforting symptoms of PMS in a number of ways. Because vegetables, whole grains, and fresh fruits are high in fiber but low in fat and sodium, they help prevent pain from constipation and bloating, common with PMS. Complex carbs can also curb cravings for sweet or salty treats, and appear to raise blood levels of tryptophan, an amino acid that converts to serotonin, the feel-good brain chemical that may modulate PMS symptoms. Consider: One study found that, compared to women who are PMS-free, women experiencing monthly symptoms consume 62 percent more refined carbohydrates (and 78 percent more sodium).

Grazing. To reduce bloating, munch on smaller, more frequent meals that spread the demands on your digestive system more evenly throughout the day.

Notable nutrients. Research suggests that women who get

more of certain vitamins and minerals have less pain and other symptoms of PMS. These include:

➤ **Calcium.** A study of 500 women found that taking 300 mg of chewable calcium carbonate (Tums) four times a day significantly reduced pain, bloating, back pain, food cravings, mood swings, and depression. If your diet's light on milk, yogurt, and cheese, ask your doctor about supplements.

➤ **Magnesium.** A daily dose of 200 mg of magnesium reduced fluid retention, breast tenderness, and bloating by 40 percent in another study. Some researchers suggest taking 500 to 1,000 mg of magnesium daily, starting on day 15 of your cycle and continuing until menstruation begins.

➤ **Vitamin E.** Claims for this nutrient are less conclusive, but some researchers believe it reduces cramps and breast tenderness.

Exercise. Study after study confirms that regular exercise such as brisk walking, swimming, or cycling improves overall health and sense of well-being, making it a key part of most treatment plans for chronic pain, and PMS is no exception. In one study, women who jogged 12 miles weekly for six months reported a reduction in PMS symptoms, while sedentary women didn't improve. Research also suggests that aerobic exercise reduces fluid retention and breast tenderness.

Comfortable clothing. If your breasts feel sore and tender, wear a larger-than-usual bra.

MEDICAL MEASURES

Pain relievers. PMS problems such as headache, backache, cramping, and breast tenderness can usually be relieved with nonsteroidal anti-inflammatory drugs (NSAIDs). Mark your calendar for when to take them: Studies suggest that NSAIDs best relieve PMS pain when they're started seven days before menstruation and continued for four days after your period starts. Over-the-counter medications such as ibuprofen (Advil, Motrin, Nuprin) and naproxen (Aleve) generally work well for mild symptoms, as do PMS-specific pain relievers such as Midol, Pamprin, or Premsyn, which combine acetaminophen with agents such as a diuretic or an antihistamine. If OTCs don't help, your doctor may suggest a prescription NSAID such as mefenamic acid, which studies specifically show helps relieve PMS pain, or COX-2 drugs (Celebrex, Vioxx, Bextra).

Diuretics. If bloating and fluid retention are your chief complaints, a doctor may prescribe a stand-alone diuretic such as spironolactone (Aldactone) to help eliminate water and sodium.

Hormonal therapy. By stopping ovulation and hormonal surges, hormone treatments may halt PMS pain as well. These therapies include:

➤ **Oral contraceptives.** Though not all birth control pills effectively control PMS, a new option in the U.S. holds much hope. Called Yasmin, it contains estrogen and drospirenone, which is similar to natural progesterone, as well as spironolactone, so it both suppresses ovulation and reduces water retention. Early studies suggest it's more effective than other contraceptives at improving PMS. "Yasmin also seems to be less likely to induce moodiness, which can be a side effect of some contraceptives," says Mark Nixon, M.D., assistant professor of obstetrics/gynecology at the University of Massachusetts in Worcester.

➤ **GnRH agonists.** Gonadotropin-releasing hormone agonists such as leuprolide acetate (Lupron) may help by making your body think it's hit menopause: No periods means no PMS. However, these drugs are reserved for severe cases because they can cause bone loss that leads to osteoporosis, says Nixon.

Antidepressants. For primarily emotional symptoms—the reason for which most women with PMS and PMDD seek treatment—selective serotonin reuptake inhibitor (SSRI) antidepressants may help. Research suggests that SSRIs such as fluoxetine (including Sarafem, recently approved for the treatment of PMDD) successfully reduce painful PMS symptoms in up to 70 percent of women who take them. Thanks to low doses and a short course (usually just during the week or so before menstruation) there's less risk of side effects such as insomnia, gastrointestinal problems, and drowsiness. Studies have also shown positive effects from nonselective serotonin reuptake inhibitors such as bupropion.

MORE THAN HORMONES

Most people explain PMS in a word: hormones. Researchers agree that cyclic changes in the sex hormones estrogen and progesterone may contribute to the problem—but probably aren't entirely to blame. Experts suspect that hormonal imbalances are triggers that ultimately may interfere with production of brain chemicals such as serotonin, a neurotransmitter that's important for feelings of well-being. Other possible (but unproven) influences include hormones other than the usual suspects, nutritional deficiencies, fluid and sodium retention, low blood sugar, and a heightened response to stress. Given the wide array of symptoms and individual differences in severity, it's possible that all these factors play at least some role in PMS.

COMPLEMENTARY OPTIONS

Mind/body methods. Because PMS often produces negative emotions that can make pain more difficult to deal with, some researchers contend that changing negative thinking and looking at menstruation in a more positive light can ease physical symptoms. Although study results are mixed and inconclusive, some research suggests that cognitive behavioral therapy works. In one study, women who took part in a behavioral program reported a 75 percent reduction in PMS symptoms. Studies also suggest that guided imagery, progressive muscle relaxation, and deep breathing may be valuable for coping with premenstrual pain.

Herbal options. Women interested in exploring herbal remedies have a number of options, including PMS combinations (also called "women's formulas") that offer several types of potentially helpful herbs, sometimes along with nutrients. Herbs most often touted for PMS relief include:

➤ **Evening primrose oil,** which may help reduce fluid retention, breast tenderness, and mood swings

➤ **Chasteberry** and **dong quai,** which are often taken for bloating, depression, and irritability

➤ **St. John's wort,** which studies have shown can alleviate mood swings and mild to moderate depression

Chiropractic. In one small study, spinal manipulation and soft-tissue therapy—both therapies provided by chiropractors—performed two or three weeks before menstruation seemed to reduce PMS symptoms.

Pokes and presses. Some women report that both acupuncture and acupressure relieve pain in the pelvic area when proper acupoints are stimulated either by (respectively) needles or manual pressure.

READY RESOURCES

American College of Obstetricians and Gynecologists
409 12th St. S.W.
Box 96920
Washington, D.C. 20090-6920
Phone: 800-673-8444
Website: www.acog.org

National Women's Health Information Center
8550 Arlington Blvd.
Suite 300 Fairfax, VA 22031
Phone: 800-994-9662
Website: www.4woman.gov

Good days, bad days: With rheumatoid arthritis, flare-ups tend to set the tone of life, particularly when pain and swelling make it difficult to perform even basic tasks such as buttoning a shirt or taking the stairs. But here's some good news: "There's been an explosion of new therapies for rheumatoid arthritis during the past decade, and their results have been fabulous," says Gary S. Firestein, M.D., chief of the division of rheumatology, allergy, and immunology at the University of California in San Diego. Better drugs to control RA—along with lifestyle changes that relieve pain and ease stress on aching joints—will help ensure your good days outnumber the bad.

Understanding the Pain

The experience of more than 2 million Americans (mostly women) who have rheumatoid arthritis differs in some respects from those who have the far more common osteoarthritis (see page 172). While OA typically develops slowly, RA often becomes obvious within a few months of the first mild aches and pains, and tends to hit earlier in life, usually between ages 20 and 50. Another difference: Rheumatoid arthritis is an autoimmune disease, meaning your own immune system attacks your body, mistaking healthy cells for viruses, bacteria, or other invaders. In this case, disease-fighting white blood cells turn against the lubricating synovial membranes that line joints. The result: pain, swelling, tenderness, warmth, and redness. Inflamed membranes make the problem worse by releasing enzymes that may eat away bone and cartilage, causing affected joints to lose shape, alignment, and mobility.

RA most often strikes the wrists, hands, feet, and ankles (usually on both sides of the body), but may also target the elbows,

INSTANT ACTION

■ Use splints or supports when pain is most severe.

■ Apply heating pads or cold packs, depending on which give you the most relief.

■ Smooth on a soothing heat ointment.

■ Rub out pain with self-massage.

■ Take NSAIDs at bedtime and on rising to reduce morning pain.

■ Relieve pressure on aching joints with specially designed devices and appliances.

shoulders, hips, knees, neck, and jaw. Pain isn't uniform, but instead tends to be worse in the morning and during periodic flare-ups that alternate with intervals of milder symptoms. Though concentrated in joints, RA affects the entire body, including the heart, blood vessels, lungs, and eyes, and may cause symptoms such as fever, fatigue, and loss of appetite. "But severe systemic complications are becoming increasingly rare, probably because treatment has gotten so good," says Firestein.

SELF-CARE STRATEGIES

Splints and supports. Finger and wrist splints, knee wraps, and other supportive aids help keep joints immobile during flare-ups, reducing pain by taking pressure off hard-working joints. Don't wear a splint nonstop, however: Keeping joints immobile for long periods can cause them to become even stiffer and surrounding muscles weaker.

Heat, cold, or both. Warmth from a hot-water bottle, steamy bath, shower, heating pad, or (for hand pain) a specially designed mitt can ease pain and increase flexibility, probably by boosting blood flow to joints. Some people, however, seem to get more relief from applying an ice pack, which numbs the nerves around inflamed joints. For the best of both worlds, alternately soak aching joints in warm water for 10 minutes, then in cold water for one minute. Repeat two more times, ending with another warm dunk—a process that works especially well for hands and feet.

Paraffin wax. Paraffin treatments, a popular spa indulgence, provide tangible benefits as therapy for RA: When hands are dipped in the hot wax, the soothing heat penetrates into aching joints. Chiropractors, massage therapists, and physical therapists offer the treatment, but you can also buy kits over the counter at drugstores and medical-supply stores.

Do-it-yourself massage. Warmed-up joints will feel even better if you take a few moments to gently stroke and press them, perhaps using a massage appliance. Although self-massage isn't difficult, the Arthritis Foundation suggests consulting a massage therapist who can offer specific advice on easing your particular pain.

Joint-saving moves. Whenever possible, use healthy parts

CHECKLIST FOR RELIEF

✔ Self-Care Strategies

Splints and supports

Heat and cold — p. 88

Contrast baths — p. 88

Paraffin wax

Self-massage

Joint-saving devices

Green tea

Strength training — p.106

Aerobic exercise — p.104

✔ Medical Measures

Pain-relieving ointments — p. 49

NSAIDs — p. 41

DMARDs

Biologic response modifiers

Corticosteroids — p. 44

Prosorba

Surgery

✔ Complementary Options

Fish oil

Gamma-linolenic acid

Boswellia — p.125

Devil's claw — p.125

Turmeric (curcumin) — p.127

Acupuncture — p.113

T'ai chi — p. 97

Yoga — p. 96

Biofeedback — p. 79

Deep breathing — p. 71

Progressive muscle relaxation — p. 77

of your body to reduce pressure on RA-afflicted joints. For example, use your hip to close doors or your palm to press the buttons on a phone. (You may want to buy a phone with over-size buttons.)

Helpful devices. In addition to big-button phones, a wide array of joint-friendly devices and appliances can ease pain caused by grabbing, twisting, and bending. Among them: long-handled toothbrushes and electric razors, easy-to-grip cook-ware, doorknob turners, raised toilet seats, and extra-graspable beverage holders. To find suppliers, check out an online resource such as www.arthritis.com (click on Assistive Products).

Green tea. Researchers say drinking about four cups of green tea a day may reduce the pain and overall severity of RA—probably due to green tea's polyphenols, powerful antioxidants that appear to reduce joint inflammation.

Exercise. With RA, the overactive immune system tends to boost metabolism, which can cause the body to burn muscle. But you can reverse muscle loss if you do resistance training, according to Tufts University researchers. In studies, the researchers found that RA patients who built stronger muscles reduced their pain by 43 percent and improved their ability to perform a range of physical functions such as walking, sitting, or tying shoelaces. Other research finds that aerobic exercise can also relieve inflamed joints.

MEDICAL MEASURES

Pain-relieving ointments. Rubbing a cream that contains capsaicin may relieve aching joints by triggering the release of endorphins, brain chemicals that provide pain relief. Although research reveals that capsaicin is most beneficial for osteoarthri-tis, it's often recommended for RA as well. Other OTC heating ointments that increase blood flow, warm the skin, and soothe pain and inflammation include Ben Gay, Miracle Ice, and oil of wintergreen.

Well-timed NSAIDs. Medical treatment of RA usually begins with nonsteroidal anti-inflammatory drugs (NSAIDs)—but you can enhance their effectiveness by timing your doses. Studies suggest that the best time to take NSAIDs for RA are after supper and first thing in the morning, which cuts pain from symptoms that gradually become more severe during the night. OTC options include ibuprofen (Advil or Motrin) or naproxen (Aleve), though you may find COX-2 inhibitors (Celebrex, Vioxx, and Bextra) gentler on the stomach.

Disease modifiers. The second-line defense against RA consists of disease-modifying antirheumatic drugs (DMARDs) such as methotrexate (Rheumatrex) and sulfasalazine (Azulfidine), which keep pain in check by slowing progression of the disease. DMARDs appear to correct joint-destroying immune-system abnormalities that cause RA, though it can take up to eight months to notice their effects. New DMARDs continue to be developed: Two European studies found that a new drug called leflunomide (Arava) may work even better than sulfasalazine. Older, traditional choices include gold salts and hydroxychloroquine (Placquenil), an antimalarial drug, which is thought to reduce the autoimmune response and lesson mild to moderate symptoms. Whatever form you use, DMARDs require close monitoring because they may cause serious side effects, including liver damage.

> ## A COURSE FOR COPING
>
> For many patients, dealing with arthritis means coping with a cycle of pain, depression, and stress. To help people take better charge of their care and comfort, the Arthritis Foundation teaches the Arthritis Self-Help Course through local offices. The 12- to 15-hour program, developed by the Multipurpose Arthritis and Musculoskeletal Diseases Center at Stanford University, offers a wealth of information about rheumatoid arthritis (as well as osteoarthritis), exercise, nutrition, pain management, medication, and nontraditional treatments. For information, contact the Arthritis Foundation.

New-generation drugs. In 1999, another class of drugs joined the anti-RA arsenal: biologic response modifiers, or BRMs, which target specific components of the autoimmune response. Some drugs in this category, such as etanercept (Enbrel) and infliximab (Remicade), lower levels of tumor necrosis factor (TNF), a protein produced by the immune system that appears both to cause inflammation and destroy joints. In one study, 70 percent of RA patients who used etanercept had less pain and swelling—and almost one-quarter reported 100 percent improvement. Another BRM called anakinra (Kineret) inhibits interleukin-1, a different inflammation-causing protein.

Corticosteroids. If your joints are sore and swollen despite RA-targeting drugs, your doctor may prescribe corticosteriods, which provide relief both by blocking the body's ability to make substances that cause inflammation and slowing autoimmune activity. Though once touted as an arthritis cure, steroids have fallen from favor due to side effects such as bone loss, cataracts, and increased risk of infection. Today, corticosteroids are generally given as low-dose pills or occasional injections into joints (three to four times yearly). They're particularly useful for "bridging" therapy—providing temporary relief while you wait for slow-acting DMARDs to take effect.

Blood wash. A new procedure called Prosorba, which absorbs antibodies from blood, offers another option if you have severe RA. Sometimes described as "washing the blood," the treatment is similar to dialysis: Blood is drawn, passed through a glass column where certain antibodies are removed, and returned to the body. It's difficult and expensive, but may help reduce pain that can't be controlled with other therapies.

Physical and occupational therapy. Whirlpool baths, ultrasound, and hot and cold packs offered by physical therapists can ease pain, while range-of-motion exercises can help keep joint mobility and function. Occupational therapists can help disabled patients learn to perform day-to-day tasks in new ways that allow them to be self-sufficient.

Possible procedures. If pain and stiffness continue to disrupt your life despite arthritis-fighting drugs and lifestyle changes, consider consulting an orthopedic surgeon. Common operations for RA include:

➤ **Arthroplasty,** also known as total joint replacement, in which artificial implants replace poorly functioning joints

➤ **Arthroscopy,** or taking out bits of bone and cartilage that cause pain and inflammation

➤ **Osteotomy,** or reshaping the damaged joint (common for knees)

➤ **Synovectomy,** or removing the diseased joint lining (common for wrists)

COMPLEMENTARY OPTIONS

Fish oil. A wealth of studies show that fish oil reduces the pain and inflammation of RA, thanks to the omega-3 fatty acids it contains, particularly eicosapentaenoic acid (EPA) and docosahexaenoic acid (DHA). Fatty acids spur production of prostaglandins, compounds that suppress inflammation and thereby dull pain. In some studies, participants have taken sizable daily doses of EPA and DHA, but you may get some benefit from as little as three weekly servings of cold-water fish, such as salmon, whitefish, and mackerel.

Gamma-linolenic acid. Another potentially helpful, inflammation-fighting fatty acid, called gamma-linolenic acid (GLA), is found in evening primrose oil. In one study, taking GLA supplements relieved RA pain enough after a year to allow subjects to lower their NSAID dosages. Currant-seed and borage oils appear to offer similar benefits. Check with your doctor before using GLA, as these oils can thin the blood and decrease its ability to clot.

Herbal options. A few herbs hold particular promise for RA, including:

➤ **Boswellia,** which in one study relieved symptoms as effectively as oral gold salts

➤ **Devil's claw,** which appears to reduce pain and improve mobility

➤ **Curcumin,** an extract of turmeric, which seems to have anti-inflammatory properties and has produced promising results in preliminary studies

Needle treatment. Early evidence suggests that acupuncture can relieve the pain of arthritis, according to the National Institutes of Health.

Mind/body moves. T'ai chi and yoga, exercises that gently work muscles and joints while encouraging relaxation through breathing and focus, help you condition your body so it's less prone to pain—and they boost your mood.

Mental methods. In one study, improvements from using behavior-modification therapies such as biofeedback allowed RA patients to reduce their clinic visits, spend less time in hospitals, and cut their medical costs. Researchers also say that relaxation techniques such as deep breathing and progressive muscle relaxation (in which you tense and release muscles one at a time) also appear to relieve pain and anxiety related to RA.

READY RESOURCES

American College of Rheumatology
1800 Century Place
Suite 250
Atlanta, GA 30345
Phone: 404-633-3777
Fax: 404-633-1870
Website: www.rheumatology.org

Arthritis Foundation
P.O. Box 7669
Atlanta, GA 30357-0669
Phone: 800-283-7800
Website: www.arthritis.org

Johns Hopkins Arthritis
Johns Hopkins University
Division of Rheumatology
Website: www.hopkins-arthritis.som.jhmi.edu

National Institute of Arthritis and Musculoskeletal and Skin Diseases
National Institutes of Health
One AMS Circle
Bethesda, MD 20892-3675
Phone: 877-226-4267
Fax: 301-718-6366
Website: www.niams.nih.gov

J ust try saying "temporomandibular joint disorders" five times fast—an especially challenging task when pain in your jaw makes it difficult to open and close your mouth. An estimated 10 million Americans, mostly women, are plagued by some form of painful trouble in the jaw's hinge-like temporomandibular joint. The problems don't always last long: About 80 percent of cases involving the joint resolve naturally within six months. But you can speed pain relief and, ultimately, recovery through self-care measures such as taking common over-the-counter medications and adjusting habitual ways you use your jaw, or taking advantage of a variety of medical treatments.

Understanding the Pain

Compared to other joints, the jaw is a very sophisticated machine—a complex, hardworking network of muscles, ligaments, bones, and teeth that can move in multiple directions to allow us to speak, chew, swallow, and show facial expression. Up, down, back, forward, side to side—all of these movements hinge on the temporomandibular joint, which connects the lower jaw, or mandible, to the temporal bone at the side of the head. A soft, shock-absorbing disk of cartilage that lies between the temporal bone and the lower jaw's rounded end helps keep the motion smooth.

Though the system usually works without a hitch, it's vulnerable to a variety of assaults that cause pain and make it difficult to use the jaw. Sometimes called TMJ but known collectively as temporomandibular disorders (TMD), common symptoms include pain when yawning, chewing, or talking; clicking or popping noises as the mouth opens and closes; tender facial muscles; a stuck or locked jaw; earache; headache; neck and shoulder pain; dizziness; and hearing problems. Frequent causes of TMD pain include:

INSTANT ACTION

■ Start with a nonsteroidal anti-inflammatory drug to minimize muscle aches and inhibit inflammation.

■ Take a prescription muscle relaxant.

■ Wear a bite plate to reduce pain from grinding.

■ Indulge in deep breathing to quickly calm tense muscles and reduce stress.

■ Eliminate pain at the source by avoiding habits such as chewing pencils or resting your jaw in your hand.

Stress and strain. Repeatedly clenching the jaws or grinding your teeth strains muscles and can eventually cause spasms typical of TMD. Psychological stress is a probable trigger, though it's unclear whether feeling personal strain causes pain or vice-versa. This type of pain usually takes the form of a cramping, aching, or burning feeling that gets worse the more the jaw is used. While usually making the chewing muscles feel tender, pain can also radiate to the neck and shoulders.

Injury. It doesn't take a heavy blow to the jaw to do damage: Even vigorous chewing or an extra wide yawn can cause pain by displacing the cushioning cartilage disks of the jaw joint. Often, displaced disks simply slip back into place, but if dislocation occurs repeatedly, the jaw may start working less smoothly and start to click, pop, and hurt whenever opened, in some cases locking into place.

Arthritis. Rheumatoid or osteoarthritis may cause the jaw joints to degenerate, leading to inflammation, stiffness, and pain. Although some researchers believe that a bad bite or poor orthodontic treatment may cause TMD, recent studies dispute these ideas, according to the National Institute of Dental and Craniofacial Research (NIDCR).

SELF-CARE STRATEGIES

Physical treatments. Applying heat from a warm compress or hot-water bottle can ease pain by relaxing sore muscles, while using cold from an ice pack to cool the hinge of the jaw can reduce discomfort from joint inflammation. Also try performing a gentle massage of sore spots around the jaws, neck, eyes, and ears to soothe tension and pain.

NSAIDs. Try over-the-counter nonsteroidal anti-inflammatory drugs like aspirin, ibuprofen, or naproxen to relieve pain and reduce inflammation.

Rest. The most important way to quell pain is to take control of what's causing it. Give your jawbones a rest, avoiding big yawns, exuberant singing or shouting, extended conversations—anything that requires the jaw to open wide or work hard. In many cases, habits you're not even aware of can contribute to pain. For example, guard against unconsciously chewing pencils or biting your nails.

CHECKLIST FOR RELIEF

✔ Self-Care Strategies

Heat and cold	p. 88
Rest	
Avoiding hard-to-chew foods	
Gentle jaw exercises	

✔ Medical Measures

Muscle relaxants	
Bite plate	
Spray and stretch	
Diathermy	
NSAIDs	p. 41
Corticosteroids	p. 44
Surgery	

✔ Complementary Options

Relaxation	p. 76
TENS	p.102
Alexander Technique	p. 98

Ailments

EASING PAIN WITH POSTURE

If you suffer from TMD, straighten up—better posture may help relieve pain in the jaw. Researchers in Texas recently separated chronic TMD patients into one group that received only symptom-management instructions (such as resting muscles, applying heat and cold, and using NSAIDs), and another group that received the same tips along with posture training focused on the head and neck. Those who got the posture pointers reported, on average, a 42 percent reduction of pain and other TMD symptoms, compared with only 8 percent less pain for those who learned symptom management only. Other research suggests that improving overall posture reduces strain on the jaw. Posture practices to avoid include:

- Resting your chin in your hand
- Reading in bed with your neck bent
- Cradling a phone with your head and shoulder
- Slouching on a sofa
- Sleeping on your stomach

Dietary protection. You can hardly avoid chewing if you want to eat. But steer clear of hard, sticky, or chewy foods, such as carrots, apples, steak, bagels, and chewing gum. During times of acute pain, consider adhering to a soft or even liquid diet for a day or two. And never bite off more than you can chew: If you can't resist a Dagwood-size sandwich piled high with fixings, squish it down to a bite-size level before you open wide and sink your teeth into it.

Gentle exercises. A number of simple moves can gently stretch or strengthen the jaw, keep you from clenching, or relax muscles. For example:

➤ Rest the front of your tongue on the roof of your mouth, with your teeth slightly parted but your lips closed.

➤ With your tongue still in place, try gently opening and closing your mouth, or moving your jaw gently from side to side.

MEDICAL MEASURES

Muscle relaxants. If muscle strain and spasms are behind the pain, a dentist or physician may prescribe a muscle relaxant such as diazepam (Valium). "These medications help break the cycle of grinding and subsequent inflammation," says David A. Bresler, D.D.S., associate professor at Temple University School of Dentistry in Philadelphia.

Bite plate. A plastic guard that fits over the upper and lower teeth may reduce the clenching or grinding and relax tense, aching jaw muscles. The guard, also known as a bite plate or splint, is usually worn at night but can also be used during the day.

Physical therapy. A physical therapist can help guide you through a variety of techniques and treatments to help control TMD, including exercises that require expert monitoring (such as some forms of neck stretches) and diathermy, a process in which an electrical current is used to generate relaxing heat deep within the muscles. Another technique often performed by physical therapists is called spray and stretch. It involves spraying the face with a numbing coolant to ease pain and relax the jaw muscles, which can then be stretched without causing discomfort.

NSAIDs. Inflammation or injury in the joints may call for a prescription NSAID such as Celebrex and Vioxx (common treatments for arthritis) to relieve pain and swelling.

Steroids. For severe inflammation, steroids might be injected into the joint, though concern about side effects generally limits their use.

Surgery. Occasionally, surgery may be recommended for an arthritic joint or injured jaw, but this should be reserved only for severe cases. According to the NIDCR, replacing jaw joints with artificial implants may cause even greater pain and lead to permanent damage, as some devices fail to work properly or may break apart over time. If surgery is suggested, be sure to seek a second opinion.

COMPLEMENTARY OPTIONS

Relaxation. Because of TMD's connection with stress, relaxation techniques may go a long way toward relieving pain. For example, many people report success using biofeedback to relax tension throughout the body—especially, in this case, chronically tensed muscles in the jaw. Another favorite of TMD doctors is deep breathing, which both helps muscles relax and turns your mind away from pain.

TENS. Some TMD sufferers report that transcutaneous electrical nerve stimulation, or applying small amounts of electrical current to joints, can help alleviate jaw pain, though studies of the method tend to produce inconsistent results.

Movement therapy. Building on the idea that posture can affect the amount of strain on the jaw and influence how it moves, posture-correcting movement therapies such as the Alexander Technique are sometimes recommended for improving muscle control and easing pain. Yoga, t'ai chi, and almost any kind of dance classes also help improve posture.

READY RESOURCES

American Academy of Otolaryngology-Head and Neck Surgery
One Prince St.
Alexandria, VA 22314-3357
Phone: 703-836-4444
Fax: 703-519-1587
Website: www.entnet.org

National Institute of Dental and Craniofacial Research
National Institutes of Health
Bethesda, MD 20892-2190
Phone: 301-496-4261
Website: www.nidcr.nih.gov

The TMJ Association
P.O. Box 26770
Milwaukee, WI 53226
Fax: 414-259-8112
Website: www.tmj.org

When you feel the heat of the sun on your face, nurse a nose that's raw from blowing, chew a savory chocolate, or bundle a scarf around your chin against a brisk winter wind, you're responding to signals carried by the trigeminal nerve—a thoroughfare of sensation with several branches to different areas of the face. When you develop trigeminal neuralgia (also called tic douloureux or tic douloureitrux), the same nerve can be the source of sudden onslaughts of intense facial pain. But even though much about trigeminal neuralgia is mysterious, doctors have come up with a number of remarkable procedures that can turn the pain off—assuming that readily available drugs haven't solved the problem first.

Understanding the Pain

Although trigeminal neuralgia is sometimes secondary to another condition, such as multiple sclerosis or a tumor or an aneurism pressing on the nerve, the disorder's cause is usually a mystery. Pain from trigeminal neuralgia can be triggered by a variety of seemingly innocuous activities, such as talking, chewing, swallowing, brushing teeth, or putting on makeup—a reflection of the fact that the condition is more common in women than men, for unknown reasons, although hormones are suspected. It's also most common after age 50, and is more likely to occur with advancing years, though cases have been seen in all age groups. Trigeminal neuralgia can appear to go into remission for periods lasting weeks, months, or even years, but the pain invariably returns.

People with trigeminal neuralgia often describe attacks as the worst pain they've ever experienced. There's no doubt trigeminal neuralgia is extraordinarily intense. The pain often occurs on one side of the face in bouts that come

INSTANT ACTION

■ Stay indoors in cold weather if facial nerves seem sensitive to low temperatures.

■ If you go outside, wear a scarf.

■ Rub in an ointment containing capsaicin.

■ Keep a pain diary to detect any patterns in flare-ups that might help you plan daily activities.

■ Stay active. Fear of pain can keep you at home and isolated, but psychologists who treat trigeminal neuralgia say you'll cope better by getting out as much as possible.

on suddenly, last a matter of seconds or minutes, then just as suddenly go away. A fresh attack often follows soon after, with some victims suffering as many as 100 episodes a day. Each attack is intense enough to incapacitate sufferers, and the on-again, off-again bouts can last for weeks or months at a time. Over time a continuous dull ache or burning sensation may occur in the affected area between the more instense attacks.

Placating the Pain

Despite its mysterious origins, doctors are gaining insights about trigeminal neuralgia that may lead to successful treatment for some patients. For example, there's evidence that some cases are caused when blood vessels grow too near the trigeminal nerve and put pressure on it, a problem that may be corrected with surgery.

SELF-CARE STRATEGIES

Sidestep triggers. Since the underlying problems leading to trigeminal neuralgia still aren't well understood, it's difficult to say how the disorder might be best prevented or minimized. The wisest bet outside of medical treatment may be to identify whatever seems most likely to trigger an attack, and avoid doing it. Many sufferers, for example, find that their pain is sensitive to cold, and therefore they try to stay indoors when it's chilly or breezy, or, when they do go out, they wear warm scarves to protect their faces.

Try a hot ointment. Some people find a measure of relief from over-the-counter ointments containing capsaicin, an irritating compound found in hot chilies that's sometimes effective against neurological pain. Take care not to get the substance too close to the eyes, however.

Practical help. If eating seems to instigate painful episodes at times, ask your doctor or a nutritionist about sipping high-nutrition liquid meals such as Encore or taking other supplements in lieu of regular food.

MEDICAL MEASURES

Adjuvant drugs. Treatment for trigeminal neuralgia usually begins with antiseizure drugs such as carbamazepine (Tegretol,

Carbatrol)—drugs that provide some measure of control over attacks in as many as 80 percent of cases, though their effectiveness diminishes the more you use them. Other anti-convulsant drugs that may be effective include phenytoin (Dilantin, Phenytex), which is sometimes combined with carbamazepine; gabapentin (Neurontin), and oxcarbazepine (Trileptal). Antidepressants may be tried as well, along with baclofen (Lioresal), a muscle relaxant that's sometimes taken in tandem with the anticonvulsant carbamazepine. Newer opioids, often combined with other drugs, such as nonsteroidal anti-inflammatory drugs (NSAIDs) like aspirin, ibuproven, or naproxen, are proving more effective in trials than more established opiods were before.

Nerve neutralizers. If drugs don't work, doctors may be able to relieve the electrifying shocks of facial pain using a variety of other techniques designed to damage or neutralize portions of the trigeminal nerve that appear to be causing the agony. For example, injections of alcohol or glycerol at trigger points can provide at least temporary relief, although the pain often returns later.

Possible procedures. A variety of more involved procedures are available as well. One is to insert a hollow needle into the face through which doctors can thread a small balloon that stills the nerve by putting pressure on it when inflated (percutaneous balloon compression). A similar procedure (percutaneous stereotactic radiofrequency thermal rhizotomy) also uses a needle, but places an electrode near the nerve, which is then damaged by heat. Other techniques include gamma knife radiosurgery, in which the nerve's root is bathed in high doses of radiation—a procedure that can be done without anesthesia—and cutting the trigeminal nerve surgically.

Nerve-sparing surgery. One of the most promising procedures relieves pain while leaving the nerve alone. Called microvascular decompression, this approach involves making an incision behind the ear on the side where pain occurs, locating the trigeminal nerve, and removing or repositioning blood vessels that are pressing on it. In some cases, a small piece of padding is placed between the nerve and blood vessel to keep them from touching again. One advantage to the operation is that it spares patients the facial numbness that's often a side effect of nerve-damaging procedures.

COMPLEMENTARY OPTIONS

Acupuncture. As with other types of nerve-related pain, acupuncture can help relieve the agony of trigeminal neuralgia for some patients. Although Chinese practitioners claim that acupuncture relieves facial pain in some 70 percent of cases, this statistic is viewed with skepticism in the West. Acupuncture's effectiveness for treating trigeminal neuralgia has not been well documented here. Doctors suggest that if you have received no relief after six or more treatments, it is unlikely that acupuncture is going to help you.

Hypnosis. Some patients, who are suseptible to it, also report getting some measure of relief from hypnosis.

Meditation. To relieve the stress brought on by the electrifying pain of trigeminal neuralgis, meditation can have a calming and relaxing effect, according to the Trigeminal Neuralgia Association.

Chiropractic. Chiropractic adjustment, according to the Trigeminal Neuralgia Association, can also relieve pain in some patients.

READY RESOURCES

National Institute of Neurological Disorders and Stroke
P.O. Box 5801
Bethesda, MD 20824
Phone: 800-352-9424
Website: www.ninds.nih.gov

Trigeminal Neuralgia Association
2801 S.W. Archer Rd.
Suite C
Gainesville, FL 32608
Phone: 904-779-0333
Fax: 904-779-7681
Website: www.tna-support.org

GLOSSARY

Acetaminophen
an over-the-counter pain-relieving drug (e.g., Tylenol) that's gentler on the stomach than many other analgesics.

Acupuncture
an ancient Chinese healing technique in which fine needles are inserted at specific points in the body to cause healing or relieve pain.

Acute pain
short-lived pain that results from some form of insult to the body such as an injury, surgery, or infection.

Addiction
see "Drug addiction."

Alexander Technique
a posture-control therapy that may reduce pain by teaching you to move your body in new ways.

Analgesic
a pain-relieving drug or treatment.

Anesthesia
loss of sensation from drugs or other treatments.

Anticonvulsants
a group of drugs that prevent seizures and can help relieve certain kinds of pain.

Antidepressants
drugs used to treat depression. Some antidepressants, particularly tricyclics, are also potent tools for easing pain.

Aromatherapy
the use of aromatic oils (either inhaled or massaged into the skin) to ease pain or promote healing.

Bextra
brand name for valdecoxib, a COX-2 enzyme inhibitor introduced in 2002.

Biofeedback
a technique in which you mentally control body functions such as heart rate and muscle tension by monitoring readouts of your physical responses.

Body scan
systematic concentration on various parts of your body to discover areas of tension and make muscles relax.

Botox
a powerful toxin that, when injected in small amounts, can block pain signals to muscles.

Breakthrough pain
pain that flares up despite your taking pain-relieving medication, often making an additional dose of medication necessary.

Capsaicin
a pepper-based substance that can interfere with pain signals when rubbed on the skin.

Celebrex
brand name for celecoxib, a COX-2 enzyme inhibitor.

Cerebral cortex
a part of the brain considered the seat of higher thinking. The cerebral cortex evaluates and interprets pain signals throughout the body and helps govern the body's response.

Chiropractor
a specialist who believes pain and other conditions can be relieved by correcting misalignments in the spine.

Chondroitin sulfate
a natural component of cartilage that, when taken as a supplement, may ease pain from osteoarthritis.

Chronic pain
longstanding persistent pain, generally defined as lasting six months or longer. Unlike acute pain, it may not have a clear cause and its exact location may be difficult to pinpoint.

Corticosteroids
hormone-like drugs that reduce inflammation and pain, but are often used only for short periods to stave off severe side effects.

COX-2 enzyme inhibitors
nonsteroidal anti-inflammatory drugs that suppress enzymes contributing to pain, but have little effect on enzymes that protect the stomach.

Deep breathing
a relaxation technique in which drawing air deep into the lungs calms the mind and produces a range of physical effects, such as reducing muscle tension and lowering blood pressure.

Dependence
see "Drug dependence."

Distraction
taking your mind off pain by concentrating on sensations, ideas, or activities that are pleasant or engaging.

Drug addiction
compulsive use of a drug to satisfy a psychological craving even when it may hurt your health, as opposed to deliberate use of the drug to meet a medical need.

Drug dependence
physical adaptation to the use of a drug so that lack of it will cause withdrawal symptoms.

Drug tolerance
the body's adjustment to a drug so that it causes fewer side effects and becomes less effective.

Endorphins
natural morphine-like painkillers the body produces on its own.

Ether
a colorless gas that was one of the first known anesthetics.

Gate control theory
the idea that pain impulses pass through a number of chemical junctures, or "gates," which may be closed to pain when the nervous system uses the same gates for other types of signals.

Glucosamine
a molecule related to sugar that's a building block of cartilage. Taken as a supplement, glucosamine may relieve pain from osteoarthritis and help repair deteriorating joints.

Histamine
a chemical that plays a role in pain by contributing to inflammation.

Homeopathy
an alternative therapy said to stimulate the healing of painful ailments when patients take condition-specific substances in extremely diluted form.

Hydrotherapy
the use of water to relieve pain through whirlpools, showers, compresses, steam, and other methods.

Hyperalgesia
exaggerated sensitivity to pain that can make even the slightest touch feel excruciating.

Hypnosis
a still-mysterious process in which susceptible people may relieve pain by going into a trance-like state.

Imagery
a technique (also known as visualization) in which you force pain from your mind by taking yourself on a mental journey or imagining a highly specific scenario.

Inflammation
a natural reaction to various forms of damage to the body that typically results in swelling and pain.

Injection therapy
rapid delivery of drugs to the body through needles into the nerves, spine, muscles, skin, or site of pain, often in lower doses than are necessary with drugs taken orally.

Intermittent pain
pain that comes and goes, or varies in intensity.

JCAHO
the Joint Commission on the Accreditation of Healthcare Organizations, the main healthcare certifying organization in the U.S., which recently established new guidelines for pain management.

Limbic system
a group of structures in the brain that govern emotion and play a role in personal interpretation of pain.

Magnet therapy
the use of magnets, often worn or placed in bedding or car seats, to alter magnetic fields in the body, which some people claim relieves pain.

Massage
physical manipulation of the body by a therapist who strokes, kneads, drums, or applies pressure to the body.

McGill Pain Questionnaire
a widely used assessment that helps patients describe the character as well as the intensity of their pain.

GLOSSARY

Meditation
a method for calming mind and body that typically entails deep breathing and focusing on a simple but meaningful word or phrase.

Modulation
the process in which the brain tries to change the body's response to pain by, for example, releasing endorphins.

Motor nerves
large nerves that govern the movement of muscles and quickly react to acute pain.

Musculoskeletal pain
pain in the muscles, bones, and joints, including arthritis, low-back pain, neck pain, headaches, and fibromyalgia.

Myofascial pain
pain arising from muscles or the tough tissue surrounding them.

Narcotics
a common term for opioids. Doctors prefer avoiding the term in a medical context because it's also used to describe illegal street drugs.

Neuroablation
the destruction of pain-producing nerves by freezing or burning.

Neuropathic pain
pain caused by damage to the nervous system.

Nociceptors
specialized nerve endings that receive pain signals and send them to the brain, a process known as nociception.

Non-steroidal anti-inflammatory drugs (NSAIDs)
pain relievers such as aspirin, ibuprofen, ketoprofen, naproxen, and a variety of prescription medications that work by blocking production of prostaglandins, hormone-like substances that cause inflammation.

Opioids
powerful pain relievers that are derived from the opium plant or chemically made to mimic opium's natural properties.

Osteopath
a specialist with the equivalent of a medical degree who uses spinal manipulation to correct mechanical defects that can cause pain.

Pain assessment
an evaluation that helps doctors understand how intense your pain is and what it feels like, often using rating scales or questionnaires.

Pain diary
a daily record of when and how intensely you experience pain that can help guide diagnosis and treatment.

Pain threshold
the point at which a painful sensation first becomes uncomfortable.

Pain tolerance
the amount of pain sensation you can take before it becomes unbearable.

Patient-controlled analgesia (PCA)
a method that lets patients give themselves doses of pain-relieving medication at times and in amounts they feel are right for them, usually through a wearable device.

Perception
the process by which the brain registers and interprets pain signals.

Peripheral nerves
nerves that carry signals between the central nervous system and the rest of the body.

Phantom pain
pain that feels as if it's coming from a part of the body that isn't really there due to amputation or removal.

Physical therapy
treatment designed to reduce pain and improve function through exercise, stretching, movement, heat and cold, massage, and other non-invasive, non-drug techniques.

Placebo effect
reaction to a dummy treatment that makes some people feel better due to the power of suggestion.

Progressive muscle relaxation
a technique in which you systematically tense muscles, then relax them, leaving them less tight than when you started.

Prostaglandins
hormone-like chemicals whose many powerful effects include stimulating inflammation. Anti-inflammatory drugs such as aspirin and ibuprofen ease pain by inhibiting prostaglandins.

Reflexology
an alternative therapy said to ease pain and promote healing through stimulation of the feet.

Reiki
a therapy whose practitioners claim to relieve pain by placing hands on or near specific positions to balance the body's so-called energy centers.

Relaxation therapy
treatment using a variety of techniques to calm the body and mind. These include body scan, progressive muscle relaxation, and deep breathing

SAMe
S-adenosylmethionine, a natural component of cells that may help relieve arthritis pain and repair damaged joints.

Sensitization
a process in which nerves progressively become more sensitive over a larger area, making pain more intense, persistent, and widespread.

Shiatsu
a form of Japanese massage in which practitioners apply sharp pressure to specific points on the body.

Sodium channel blockers
drugs usually prescribed to correct abnormal heart rhythms that are sometimes used to correct electrical disturbances that cause pain.

Substance P
a peptide that appears to make nerves more sensitive to pain. Topical irritants such as capsaicin work by depleting substance P at the site of pain.

T'ai chi
a martial art combining deep breathing with slow and controlled movements that may help ease pain by restoring physical function and calming the mind.

TENS
transcutaneous electrical nerve stimulation, a treatment in which a small device sends weak electrical impulses into the body through electrodes, which some people find relieves pain.

Thalamus
a site deep in the brain where pain signals first register, triggering initial reflex responses such as snatching your hand from a hot stove.

Therapeutic touch
relief of pain said to be achieved through the laying on or movement of hands near the body and the interaction of purported energy fields produced by both therapist and patient.

Tolerance
see "Drug tolerance" and "Pain tolerance."

Tramadol
a drug (Ultram) that bears similarities to both opioids and tricyclic antidepressants, often used as an intermediate step between NSAIDs and narcotics.

Transduction
a kickoff process for pain in which an injury or some other form of stimulus causes nerve cells to turn on pain signals.

Transmission
the process by which pain signals from the body travel up through the nervous system to the brain.

Trigger point
a sensitive, knotted, small area in muscle that refers pain to another part of the body.

Vioxx
brand name for rofecoxib, a COX-2 enzyme inhibitor.

Visceral pain
dull, aching pain that arises from internal organs, often in the abdomen.

Vital signs
elements evaluated to determine the fundamental health of the body, traditionally consisting of respiration, pulse, temperature, and blood pressure. Pain is now considered the fifth vital sign.

Yoga
a movement therapy that combines meditative practices with gentle exercises that may reduce pain by improving physical function, reducing tension, and fostering a positive outlook.

INDEX

double-identity drugs, 48–49
genetics and, 168
insurance coverage of, 163
modern types of, 34–35
NSAIDs, 41–43
opioids, 14, 18, 26, 45–47, 48
patient reactions to, 41
side effects of, 51, 169
topical, 49–50
tramadol, 50, 175

Duloxetine, for depression, 137

Duragesic, 55

E

Effexor, for depression, 137

Elavil, for depression, 137

Elmiron, for interstitial cystitis, 212–13

Emergency causes of pain, 21

Emotional barriers
anger, 139–41
depression, 136–39
poor self-esteem, 146–48

Emotional deconditioning, with chronic pain, 30

Emotional stages of viewing pain, 66–67

Emotions, pain and, 18, 133–34

Enbrel, for rheumatoid arthritis, 167

Endometriosis, 201–5

Endorphins, pain control from, 26–27

Energy-based therapies
reflexology, 118
reiki, 119
shiatsu, 116–17
therapeutic touch, 117–18

Epidural, for delivering opioids, 54–55

Ergonomic tools, for carpal tunnel syndrome, 188–89

Ergostat, for migraines, 221

Ergotamine tartrate, for migraines, 221

Eternacept, for rheumatoid arthritis, 167

Ether, for anesthesia, 34, 35

Ethnicity, pain tolerance and, 62

Evening primrose oil, for premenstrual syndrome, 243

Exercise
aerobic, 104–5
with pain, 103–4
starting, 105–6
strength training, 106
for stress management, 71–72
for weight loss, 149

F

Feldene, 42

Fentanyl, 46, 48, 55, 184

Feverfew, for headaches, 222

Fiber
for chronic fatigue syndrome, 196
for endometriosis, 203
for irritable bowel syndrome, 215

Fibromyalgia, 104, 206–9

Fifth vital sign, pain as, 11

Fighting, effective, 144

Financial concerns, 162–63

Fish oil
for fibromyalgia, 209
for reducing inflammation, 126–27

5-HTP, for fibromyalgia, 209

Formulary drugs, 163

Fractures, compression, back pain from, 178

Function of pain, 20–22

G

Gamma-linolenic acid
for endometriosis, 205
for peripheral neuropathy, 234
for rheumatoid arthritis, 249

Gastrointestinal problems, from NSAIDs, 44

Gate control theory of pain, 27–28

Gender
carpal tunnel syndrome and, 190
pain and, 155

Genetics
pain sensitivity and, 166
research on, 167–68

Ginger, for endometriosis, 205

Glucosamine
for arthritis, 123–24, 176
for joint problems, 124

GnRH agonists
for endometriosis, 203
for premenstrual syndrome, 242

Goals
effect of pain on, 133
for pain management, 52, 165

Green tea, for rheumatoid arthritis, 246

INDEX

H

Hamstring stretch, 94
H2 blocks, for peptic ulcers, 229
Headaches, 21, 50, 218–22
Heat treatments, 88, 89–90, 91
Hellerwork, 103
Herbal therapies. *See also specific herbs*
  quality of, 112
Hip flexor stretch, 95
Homeopathy, 120
Hyalgan, for arthritis, 175
Hyaluronic acid, for arthritis, 175
Hydrocodone, 48
Hydromorphone, 46, 48
Hydrotherapy, 90–91
Hyocyamine levsin, for irritable bowel
  syndrome, 216–17
Hypnosis
  for fibromyalgia, 209
  for pain relief, 80–81
  for postherpectic neuralgia, 238
  for trigeminal neuralgia, 257

I

Ibuprofen, 42
Ice. *See* Cold treatments
Icy Hot, 50
Imagery
  for arthritis, 176
  for cancer pain, 186
  for pain relief, 74–76
Inflammation, supplements reducing, 125–27
Injection therapies
  for cancer pain, 54, 185
  for delivering narcotics, 54–55
  for trigeminal neuralgia, 256
Insurance coverage, 162–63
Intelligence, pain perception and, 27
Intermittent pain, 22
Interstitial cystitis, 210–13
Intramuscular injections, for muscle spasms,
  55
Intraspinal injections, for delivering narcotics,
  54–55
Intravenous injections, for delivering
  narcotics, 54
Irritable bowel syndrome, 214–17

J

Joint pain
  possible causes of, 21
  supplements for, 124
Joint-protecting devices, for arthritis, 173, 246

K

Kava, for anxiety, 128
Kegel exercises, for endometriosis, 202
Ketoprofen, 42

L

Laughter, for pain relief, 82
Legislation, on pain treatment, 11
Levorphanol, 48
Licofelone, as alternative to COX-2 inhibitors,
  168–69
Licorice, for peptic ulcers, 230
Lidocaine injections
  for central pain syndrome, 193
  for fibromyalgia, 208, 209
Lidocaine patch, for postherpectic neuralgia,
  236–37
Lidoderm, for postherpectic neuralgia, 236–37
Lifting, proper form for, 181
Lollipops, opioid, 55, 184
Lotronex, for irritable bowel syndrome, 216

M

Magnesium
  for fibromyalgia, 209
  for headaches, 220
  for premenstrual syndrome, 241
Magnetic resonance imaging, for revealing
  pain, 30
Magnet therapy, 121–22
  for peripheral neuropathy, 234
Malic acid, for fibromyalgia, 209
Manipulation, 101–2
  for back pain, 181
  for fibromyalgia, 209
  for neck pain, 226
  for premenstrual syndrome, 243
MAO inhibitors, for depression, 137

Photos

16 Digital Vision, **17** Reader's Digest Assoc. Inc./GID, **20** Comstock, **31** Rubberball **44** Reader's Digest Assoc. Inc. **47** PhotoLink/Photodisc/PictureQuest, **49** Suza Scalora/ PhotoDisc/PictureQuest, **63** Branson Reynolds/ IndexStock, **68** PhotoDisc, **69** Reader's Digest Assoc. Inc./GID/ Ray Moller, **71** Dynamic Graphics, **73** DigitalVision/ PictureQuest, **75** Philip Coblentz/Brand X Pictures/ PictureQuest, **76** PhotoDisc, **78** Daniel Thistlethwaite/imagesource/PictureQuest, **81** Digital-Vision/PictureQuest, **82** Stockbyte/PictureQuest, **88** PhotoDisc, **89** Corbis, **92** Daniel Thistlethwaite/imagesource/ PictureQuest, **96** Daniel Thistlethwaite/imagesource/ PictureQuest, **97** ImageState, **105** PhotoDisc, **113** Ron Chapple/ Thinkstock/ PictureQuest, **116** Corbis, **126** Nick Koudis/ PictureQuest, **127** Reader's Digest Assoc. Inc./GID/Udo Loster, **128** Reader's Digest Assoc. Inc./GID, **135** PhotoDisc, **136** PhotoDisc, **142** PhotoDisc, **145** PhotoDisc, **149** PhotoDisc, **154** Bill Crump/Brand X Pictures/ PictureQuest, **155** Rubberball, **156** Alvis Upitis/Brand X Pictures/PictureQuest, **157** PhotoDisc, **159** Corbis, **164** DigitalVision/PictureQuest

Illustrations

Medical illustrations: **25, 100-101** Duckwall Productions
Excercise illustrations: **94-95** Julie Johnson
All other illusrations including cover: Linda Frichtel